W____

GLUTEN

The Secret to Losing Belly Fat
&
Regaining Health

Get Help from the Gluten "GO-TO" Docs

Dr Frank Lanzisera

Dr Lisa Lanzisera

Lanzisera Center for Chiropractic Medicine

Lanzisera Chiropractic Medicine LLC

17 Davis Boulevard Suite 401

Tampa Florida 33606

(813) 253-2333

Copyright © 2012 Drs. Frank and Lisa Lanzisera

Photos by www.robertcrumphotography.com

ISBN: 1478199555
ISBN-13:978-1478199557

DEDICATION

This book is dedicated to our children, Keely and Keegan, who have allowed us to enjoy life to its fullest. We also want to acknowledge the many patients we have known in our 30 plus years of practice. Thank you for the honor of entrusting us with your health care.

CONTENTS

Dedication

Acknowledgments

CHAPTERS

Skype Consultations/Videoconferencing

Web Site www.WheatGlutenDocs.com

Seminars/Social Media

Intended Use Statement

It is the intent of this book to be for informational purposes only. It is the sole responsibility of the user of this information to comply with all local, state, and federal laws and practices. The content of this book is not meant as the basis for any diagnosis, treatment, or prevention of any disease. Case studies presented in this book reflect a composite of symptoms, examinations, and treatments of several patients and not one individual in each case study. These case studies are meant to serve as examples for informational purposes only and should not be used to diagnose, treat, or prevent disease in an actual person by any healthcare professional or layperson.

Notices and Disclaimers

The contents of this book are not meant to replace or augment any professional medical care. It is the sole responsibility of the user of any information in this book to determine if any action based on this information is appropriate. The authors of this book cannot be held responsible in any way, shape, or form for the information contain herein or for any inadvertent errors, nor omissions. The nutritional compounds mentioned in this book are not intended to be used by a layperson without the supervision of a licensed medical professional. The information provided in this book is not meant to be used as a replacement for conventional medical treatment. The authors recommend readers seek the advice of a licensed medical professional before implementing any and all recommendations, real or imagined, protocols, nutritional supplements, or using any information contained in this book. The Food and Drug Administration did not evaluate the information contained herein prior to publication. The nutritional advice mentioned in this book is not intended to diagnose, cure, treat, or prevent disease or any health condition.

ACKNOWLEDGMENTS

We have been extremely fortunate to know some of the most outstanding chiropractic and medical doctors of our era but the two who have made the most life-changing impressions are L. John Faye, D.C. and Webster Marxer, M.D..

 In the early 1980's, Dr. Faye was traveling across the U.S.A. talking about how a paradigm shift was occurring in health care. He lectured at colleges throughout the country citing new research from around the world. We were excited as young doctors to be able to serve our patients with a more complete understanding of how the body could fight disease and dysfunction.

Dr. Marxer, our uncle, is considered the father of predictive medicine. He was one of the first medical doctors to use a type of cardiac stress test to predict if a patient was at risk for cardiovascular disease. He then would advise smoking cessation, weight control, and nutritional supplementation. His ideas on preventing disease were decades ahead of their time. Uncle Web was instrumental in developing the healthcare protocol for the astronaut program as well. He was a very caring doctor who made house calls night or day for his patients until he retired. Naturally curious, he never stopped learning and was always excited to discover something new that could help his patients.

Now, we are at the beginning of a new paradigm shift. Our understanding of what prevents health has broadened once again. We are grateful to have known two dedicated physicians, Dr. Faye and Dr. Marxer, who set such a high standard for the rest of us.

1

The GLUTEN DECEPTION

True Story
About 5 years ago, my husband and I were driving through the farming area of southern Illinois, when he asked if the crop to our right was wheat. I looked and said "Well, it looks like wheat, but it's too short. Wheat would be twice as tall at this point in the season..." You see, I grew up helping out on my grandparents' farm where they raised the typical Midwest crops of wheat, soybean, and corn. As kids, my cousins and I could play hide- and- seek in the wheat field because the plants were as tall as us. The plants my husband pointed out were only about 2 feet tall... but they *looked* like wheat. Little did we know that while the crop was stilled called wheat, it had been altered by genetic hybridization. This started our education into the world of genetically-engineered food and the harmful effects of modern wheat and specifically, gluten.

Non-celiac wheat sensitivity is not a fad. As recently as late July, 2012, it has been confirmed as a distinct clinical condition in a double-blind and placebo-controlled study (Am Journal Gastoenterology;PMID: 22825366). The study refers to it as a **"new clinical entity"**. This means, most doctors practicing today never learned about non-celiac wheat sensitivity (NCWS) in school. With at least one in seven people being wheat or gluten

1

sensitive, it may be the most undiagnosed condition in the world today.

There are two important facts that we need to explain. The first is that the wheat we consume today is vastly different from the wheat grown in the 1950's and '60s. It tastes the same in our food but the similarity ends there. The second fact is that this modern wheat may be extremely bad for our health. This can be hard for us to wrap our heads around...this idea that our food can make us sick. We have been taught that wheat is part of a healthy diet, even told that whole wheat breads should be part of our nutrition pyramid. In our opinion, we've been taught wrong.

Discovering the effects that modern wheat has on the human body has answered a lot of questions for us as doctors. In our 30 plus years of private practice, we would wonder why certain patients did not respond well to traditional care. For example, we would send patients for blood work if we suspected thyroid disease. If the lab tests came back positive for hypothyroidism, we would refer them to an internist or endocrinologist for further examination. Sometimes, despite having their case managed with synthetic thyroid replacement medication, the patient would continue to display the symptoms of hypothyroidism including fatigue, inability to lose weight, hair loss, depression/anxiety, constipation, and body aches and pains, etc. These patients would be put into the category of "we know something is wrong, we just don't know what it is". This is very frustrating to a physician and exasperating to patients. At the time, the healthcare community was not aware of an autoimmune disorder called Hashimoto's thyroiditis which can be triggered by sensitivity to wheat.

We also would have patients with weight problems. Their diet diaries, details compiled by the patient on what they ate each day and how much, would not reveal anything to account for their excess weight. They would have toast and eggs or cereal for breakfast, a sandwich or slice of pizza for lunch, pasta for dinner.

Occasional desserts would be a piece of cake or pie. Usually, the caloric intake would be just above their target range but typically these patients would also exercise. They seemed to be carrying much more weight than could be attributed to their diet and lifestyle. Looking back, the answer is obvious – they were gorging on wheat throughout each and every day and we would bet our last nickel that all these patients were wheat gluten sensitive.

Not only is the general population unaware of the changes that wheat has undergone in the past 50 years, doctors are unprepared to diagnose the effects this wheat can be potentially causing to the human body.

Gluten is a component of wheat that has been genetically manipulated by bioengineers. It is naturally present in wheat, barley and rye grasses. Agribusiness, in their search to produce modern wheat with higher protein content, has amplified the amount of gluten in wheat by nearly 500 times. Not only is gluten more concentrated, it reacts with the body differently than gluten found in unmodified wheat. When someone is gluten sensitive it means that their body produces antibodies against gluten and that their intestines have been damaged causing "leaky gut" syndrome. "Leaky gut" syndrome is clarified later in this book.

Non-celiac wheat sensitivity (NCWS) refers to the all the components of wheat, including gluten, that react adversely with the human body. There are multiple, elemental parts of modern wheat that can produce undesirable effects. We will explore these other components in more detail in later sections...but we will tell you this, one of them is potentially more threatening to our health than gluten.

The reason everyone seems to be talking about wheat gluten sensitivity is that it appears to have triggered the development of serious health issues and the range of conditions is staggering. Celiac disease, autism, obesity, depression, ADD/ADHD, Type2 diabetes, heart disease, chronic sinusitis, cancer, fibromyalgia, migraines/headaches, skin diseases, and auto-immune disorders such as Hashimoto's thyroiditis and rheumatoid arthritis (RA), are suspected of being gluten related. An entire chapter in this book is devoted to the many conditions associated with gluten sensitivity (GS).

It is estimated, and we agree based on our clinical observations, that **99% of those people who have a problem with gluten are not currently diagnosed.**

Gluten, however, is only one component of modern wheat that is worrisome. Wheat, as is used in food manufacturing today, does not have the same genetic makeup as naturally-evolved or wild wheat, such as Einkorn wheat. There is a significant difference between modern wheat and Einkorn wheat. Einkorn has only 14 chromosomes and is almost genetically identical to the Einkorn wheat grown thousands of years ago. Modern wheat, on the other hand, has 42 chromosomes and has been altered dramatically over the past 50 years. These 42 chromosomes have the potential of producing over 1000 different proteins that we have not yet completely identified nor do we know their effects on the human body.

The modern wheat that is currently grown may be responsible for triggering **55 diseases** according to "The New England Journal of Medicine". Serious health problems, such as celiac disease, now affect a significantly greater portion of the population than in the 1950's. **It may not be a coincidence that modern wheat was first grown about 50 years ago as well.** According to a study by researchers at the Mayo Clinic, celiac disease (CD) was rare in the early 1950s and only affected about **1 in 2,500 people.** CD now affects more than 3 million people in the U.S. alone or **1 in 133 people.**

Thyroid disease has also impacted many more lives. It is estimated that as many as 1 in 5 Americans have thyroid disease now compared to about 1 in 20 just twelve years ago. Thyroid cancer cases have also increased and are one of the only cancers that continue to rise in the United States.

Gluten contains thyroid inhibiting substances called *goitrogens*. We have seen many patients over the years that display all the symptoms of hypothyroidism but do not respond well when treated with thyroid replacement hormone. The reason for this is doctors may have been treating the *symptoms* of the condition but not the main *cause* behind the hypothyroidism. Goitrogens in gluten can induce antibodies that cross-react with the thyroid gland. They can also interfere with iodine levels in the body's production of thyroid hormones. Gluten sensitivity may be one of the reasons behind the epidemic levels of thyroid conditions.

How can wheat cause so many different health problems?

This answer is both simple and complex. Let's start with the simple version.

The gastrointestinal tract plays a prominent part in our immune system. It must prevent pathogens (germs) and food that has not been broken down sufficiently from crossing through the intestines into the bloodstream and lymph system. Gluten and other factors can cause the lining of the intestines to become less tightly meshed (commonly described as "Leaky Gut"). This allows germs, cytokines, antibodies, small bits of food and more to pass into the blood and lymph system potentially causing the body to react by attacking these foreign substances. Widespread inflammation can develop as well as food allergies and autoimmune responses. So any organ, including the brain, can be affected in this scenario. The blood-brain barrier can become dysfunctional following a breakdown in the intestinal defense system. Disorders such as anxiety, depression, and "brain fog" have been linked to wheat sensitivity. Another identified disorder of NCWS is "gluten ataxia". A person with ataxia develops loss of coordination and balance. **It is not unusual for people with NCWS to display multiple symptoms involving a web of multiple organ systems.**

A more complete answer is provided in the chapter titled "What is "Leaky Gut" Syndrome?"

What is in modern wheat that makes it harmful to the human body?

Modern wheat has been altered to the point that it now barely resembles the wheat grown through the 1960's. By using aggressive hybridization methods, it has been transformed to have **a 500 fold increase in gluten content.**

To underscore the difference between a relic crop, such as Einkorn wheat, as compared to modern wheat, just look at the number of chromosomes. Einkorn wheat, which has been harvested since the late Paleolithic and early Mesolithic Ages (16,000-15,000 B.C.), has only 14 chromosomes. Its two sets of chromosomes make it a diploid wheat. While modern wheat contains 42 chromosomes and has six sets of chromosomes making it a hexaploid wheat. These 42 chromosomes, based on sheer volume and origination, are far more likely to produce undesirable proteins.

These potentially undesirable proteins have been described in the literature as "funny" and "squishy". We prefer to describe them using the analogy of *The Incredible Hulk* .Dr. Bruce Banner is the quiet, non-threatening physicist in the story. His character represents gluten found in wheat prior to advanced genetic hybridization. Most humans could at least tolerate this amoun gluten, even though there is evidence that gluten has always been a health detriment. In the story, Dr. Banner's genes become mutated after being exposed to radiation from a gamma bomb. He becomes transformed into a raging, unpredictable, green monster. Much like the Hulk, the effects of gluten from modern wheat can be widespread and unpredictable. By potentially triggering body-wide inflammation and immune system compromises, this new wheat can wreak havoc on humans. What a coincidence that both the Hulk comic book and genetically manipulated wheat emerged in the 1960's.

Besides an extraordinary amount of gluten, modern wheat also contains wheat germ agglutinin (WGA) lectin. Researchers at the University of Verona showed that WGA lectin also causes the intestinal wall to become more permeable thus allowing substances to enter the bloodstream that normally would be blocked. These unwanted substances can then set off a chain of events within the body producing the development of allergies and autoimmune reactions (Toxicol Appl Pharmacol, 2009 June). **It's ironic that the "healthier" bread, whole wheat, actually contains the highest concentration of WGA lectin** including the sprouted form.

Lectin is a type of WGA and glycoprotein. Because wheat has been hybridized for increasingly larger amounts of protein, the amount of WGA lectin has increased as well. Lectin is a blessing and a curse for the wheat plant. It repels insects and fungi for the plant so it is inherently hard for another living system to break it down. Therefore, it accumulates in tissues. To help visualize how strong WGA lectin is, imagine trying to digest a piece of vulcanized rubber... because the same disulfide bonds in this rubber are found in WGA lectin. Lectin is classified as an **anti-nutrient because it blocks absorption of nutrients in the body. It also can** inhibit digestive enzymes and interfere with the absorption of iron and zinc.

Why should I be aware of lectin in my food?

It has been hypothesized that wheat lectin is even more dangerous than gluten. WGA lectin stimulates the production of pro-inflammatory chemical messengers called cytokines. Gluten contributes to the effect these cytokines have on the permeability of the intestinal wall. WGA lectin is also suspected of being **cytotoxic** meaning that it is toxic to cells by inducing programmed cell death. There are several more scary effects of WGA lectin beyond its ability to pass through the blood-brain barrier and inhibit survival of the brain's neurons. (Proc Natl Acad Sci U S A .1988 Jan; 85(2):632-6, PMID 2448779). These effects will be explored in a later chapter.

Is there something in wheat that makes us fat?

Yes, or more accurately, *several* components in modern wheat are present that can cause weight gain. For starters, there is a complex carbohydrate called **amylopectin A** in wheat that spikes our blood sugar levels. Repeatedly raising these levels causes us to form fat deposits around the abdomen. It is important for the public to understand the significance of *where* we gain weight on our bodies. It has been shown in a recent study presented at the European Society of Cardiology conference, ESC Congress 2012, that **accumulation of fat in the mid-section has a greater risk of death than those who are obese.** Dr. Francisco Lopez-Jimenez, senior author on the study and a cardiologist with Mayo Clinic, reported "...what is new in this research is that the distribution of the fat is very important even in people with a normal weight." He went on to say about people with mid-section fat accumulation, "This group has the highest death rate, even higher than those who are considered obese..." For more information on this on-going study involving conducted by the U.S. Centers for Disease Control log on to http://www.cdc.gov/nchs/nhanes.htm/.

Belly fat can trigger pre-diabetes, diabetes, cataracts, heart disease and other conditions. It has been shown that foods with a high glycemic index lead to a fatty liver which then sets the stage for obesity, followed by pre-diabetes, then diabetes. Presently, there is a worldwide epidemic of Type 2 diabetes in our children. Obesity levels in children continue to skyrocket. Some analysts have pointed the finger at mothers who gained too much weight during pregnancy or failed to breastfeed their children. We, however, believe that wheat sensitivity can be a factor in both Type 2 Diabetes and obesity in children and adults.

Modern wheat causes weight gain three other ways. It contains gluteomorphins, goitrogens, and lectins. Gluteomorphins affect our brains by producing a craving for wheat, goitrogens affect our metabolic rate by destabilizing the thyroid gland, and lectins cause us to store more calories as fat by creating insulin resistance.

In our clinical experience, sensitivity to wheat gluten can also cause the body to retain water. Patients note that when they have been faithful to their non-gluten diet, their rings slide easily on their fingers. They find that when they do eat gluten their rings will feel tighter the next day.

How can I tell if I am eating genetically modified (GM) foods?

The Grocery Manufacturers of America estimate about 75% of what is on the shelves in American grocery stores contain at least trace amounts of GM ingredients. Chances are high that the typical consumer has ingested this type of food for years without knowing it. Here is an easy way to differentiate by looking at the **PLU labels** on fruits and vegetables:

4- Digit number is conventionally produced

5-Digit number that begins with an 8 is GM

5-Digit number that begins with 9 is organic

If a food is labeled "organic", does that mean that it is not genetically modified (GM)?

No, foods labeled with only "organic" may still be up to 30 % GM. The US and Canadian governments do not let food manufacturers label a food "100% organic" unless the food has *not* been genetically modified *or* been fed GM feed. So it stands to reason that only 100% organic- labeled food is safe from genetic modification.

Are eggs considered to be GM?

Yes, this also applies to eggs labeled "free-range", "cage- free", and "natural" which may be GM. However, eggs labeled "100% organic" should be, according to U.S. and Canadian law, void of genetic modification.

If I am gluten sensitive, does that mean that I have celiac disease?

No, you can be GS without having a full-blown case of celiac disease. Celiac disease (CD) is a lifelong, inherited autoimmune condition affecting children and adults. Those with CD have a genetic predisposition identified as HLA DQ2 or DQ8. Celiac disease, also known as celiac sprue or gluten sensitive enteropathy (GSE), affects 1 in 133 people in the United States. Celiac disease is not a food allergy but an autoimmune disease. Sufferers of CD cannot eat any gluten from all forms of wheat including durum, semolina, spelt, kamut, and faro. They also must eliminate the grains rye, barley and triticale (Celiac Disease Foundation).

Gluten sensitivity exists independently of celiac disease. CD can be diagnosed with blood tests and biopsies. Presently, there are very few doctors who consider GS when diagnosing their patients. **It is typical for a patient with GS to endure their symptoms for years before being diagnosed.**

How can a doctor help me if I am GS?

Every patient needs a complete history to be taken by a carefully listening doctor. Many times, the history -taking portion of an examination is the most important part. So think of your doctor as one big ear. He or she will be listening for clues as to what is wrong. You know your own body better than anyone; you just need someone knowledgeable to sort things out.

When a patient presents with GS-related symptoms, a doctor will perform a physical examination including a review of systems. A neurological examination will be done to determine if the central nervous system (CNS) and/or the peripheral nervous system (PNS) are involved and to what extent. The brain- based testing portion of the examination involves testing the cerebellum and cortex for imbalances. The doctor will also want to review the metabolic function of a patient. This is accomplished by lab tests and questionnaires to determine nutritional status, immune function, and hormonal functions.

Chiropractic physicians will also be able to determine if there is a spinal component affecting the patient's health. Musculoskeletal conditions need to be addressed for a well-rounded treatment plan.

By developing a diagnosis and confirming with testing, a doctor will guide the patient back to health with an individualized treatment plan. **There is no "cookbook" solution when dealing with the human body, especially one with GS.**

To give you a better understanding of how doctors can treat this condition, we have included a Case Studies section in the chapter titled "Is Your Health Condition Caused by Gluten?"

I've eaten wheat my whole life. How can I change my eating habits?

Changing to a GF diet can be challenging so expect this transformation to take determination on your part. The most important thing to remember is that you sincerely *want* to change....and you *need* to change for the sake of your health. When other members of your household become aware of just how detrimental gluten can be, they will support you...and most likely, start eating a GF diet too. We want to note that if one family member has been diagnosed with GS, there is a greater likelihood that other members are also GS. It's important to undergo testing before beginning a GF diet: first, to know if you are sensitive and second, to know if any other food sensitivities are present.

Transitioning to a GF diet is easier if you think of it as just replacing wheat products. For instance, GF pasta definitely has a different texture than that made from durum wheat but there are all kinds of varieties. Corn-based pasta can be a little chewier than rice pasta. It takes some experimenting before finding what you prefer to eat.

Changing a habit begins in the brain. Making a decision to switch to being GF actually is initiated in the frontal cortex. This is the area of the brain closest to the forehead and is where behavioral inhibition and self-discipline are wired. Most habits can be altered by focusing on one pattern. In this case, focus on when you are most likely to eat a gluten food. For instance, you always have toast with your morning eggs. Changing this habit is relatively easy. Substitute the toast with gluten-free bread, or for an even healthier choice, a bowl of fresh blueberries and strawberries.

Most habits, good and bad, are actually automatic behaviors. The brain tries to conserve energy by eliminating the need to concentrate on every one of the thousands of little decisions we make every day. A good example of this is when you are driving home and all of a sudden you realize that you have turned on your street. You weren't entirely aware that you had guided your car to where you wanted to go because you had followed that route home so many times. The brain allowed you to think of other things thus conserving energy to dwell upon other matters. Changing a habit of eating gluten foods does require the brain to use energy. This effort lessens, though, the longer you do it. You can override old habits. A 3-Step program based on research done at the Massachusetts Institute of Technology (MIT) on habits is included in Chapter 6 of this book.

If I am GS, will I ever be able to eat wheat-based foods again?

Once you have been on a GF diet for at least 6-12 months and your symptoms have abated, you may be able to try eating gluten from relic crops. The reason for this is a relic crop, such as Einkorn wheat, has only 14 chromosomes and a different gluten structure than modern wheat which has 42 chromosomes. Einkorn wheat products are sparsely available but some people with GS report being able to consume this gluten. In 2006 it was reported in the Scandinavian Journal of Gastroenterology that **Einkorn wheat** (Triticum monococcum) **did not evoke a toxic reaction** in intestinal samples taken from celiac patients. Although further study is warranted, Einkorn wheat products may be safe for gluten sensitive and possibly, celiac patients.

Some people are able to re-introduce wheat gluten from modern wheat occasionally back into their diet with little or no adverse, overt symptoms...but why would you want to? Modern wheat can affect our body not just in easily identifiable symptoms i.e. bloating, diarrhea but also covertly involving our brain to our immune system.

The awful truth is that, although we have already discussed gluten, lectin and amylopectin A as being detrimental to our health, there are over 1000 other proteins in modern wheat that may also affect us adversely....and this book does not cover genetically modified (GM) crops : soybeans, maize, and golden rice. Dr Mae-Wan Ho has stated "Genetic engineering is inherently dangerous, because it greatly expands the scope for horizontal gene transfer and recombination, precisely the processes that create new viruses and bacteria that cause disease epidemics, and trigger cancer in cells."

The most important thing to remember is that once testing positive for GS, the body must have a chance to heal before any thought of re-introducing gluten into the diet. Working with a physician to help manage GS will help in this decision. If, however, testing has determined that you carry the gene for celiac disease then you should remain gluten free for the remainder of your life.

Where can I find gluten –free recipes?

We have included over 40 recipes of our family's favorites in this book to get you started. They range from basic breakfast food to gourmet appetizers.

Most recipes can be altered substituting wheat flour and gluten-containing products with their GF versions. You will not have to forego cakes, breads and donuts but you may have to make some of them yourself. Once you become aware of which foods contain gluten, you will usually be able to substitute them with healthy alternatives.

A periodical that we highly recommend, both for its recipes and content, can be found at www.LivingWithout.com. You can download coupons from this site as well.

We want to assure you of one thing. By the time you have finished reading this book, you will have educated yourself to the point where you are confident in your knowledge to protect yourself from known health risks. We all know knowledge is power but also that change can be difficult. So we have included a 3-step program that, if followed, will help you make the necessary changes in your lifestyle. Changes stop being new at some point and become automatic. New habits of eating become easier when your health and mental attitude are improved.

Families typically start off with the one who is unwell eating the gluten-free meals while the others still consume their usual diet. Then, through several cycles of eating GF foods and eating the old diet, the whole family moves towards the healthier eating habits. Our family has found that most recipes can be made without gluten and our favorites are included within this book. Hope you enjoy!

2

GLUTEN MEANS GLUE

Gluten is the Latin word for glue. This is an appropriate term as it is a sticky protein composite derived from wheat and other grains including barley and rye. You will note that throughout this book we refer to gluten as being *wheat* gluten. The reason for this is because some individuals who are wheat gluten sensitive are not sensitive to the gluten in barley and rye.

Wheat gluten is very common in the Western diet and is found primarily in breads, cereals, crackers and pastas. It is also found in items that you would not initially suspect such as soy sauce, some lunch meats, and….this is really going to surprise you….envelope adhesive. Even everyday condiments like ketchup and mustard can have gluten in them. It's incredible how pervasive gluten is and even a "healthy" diet can still be loaded with it. Becoming a food label detective will be one of the first steps you take to becoming healthier.

Within this book you will learn how to readily determine which foods to avoid. Living a life free of gluten is challenging at first, but, as with all habits, it will become easier. Eating out at restaurants is becoming less of a burden as that industry strives to accommodate their patrons' needs. It still is a good idea to call a restaurant beforehand to see if they can prepare gluten-free (GF) meals and it also would be prudent to ask if they use dedicated utensils when making the food to avoid cross contamination. Grocery stores have made efforts to help identify which of their thousands of products are GF. Some stores place tags under the items on the shelf to make finding their location easier for the consumer while others have whole sections dedicated to GF products. Typically, a greater selection can be found at large health-oriented stores like Whole Foods Market. Given that 1 in 7 people worldwide are gluten sensitive, it's simply good business for food manufacturers to offer GF foods in their product lines. Costs of GF foods are still on the high-end but there is now more variety. Remember, your health is well worth the time and effort.

GS causes a wide range of symptomatology. Although it can have the potential to trigger a broad spectrum of disorders, many doctors do not include it in their differential diagnosis. Especially when traditional treatments fail to render positive results, patients should request that GS tests be performed by a doctor familiar with administering them. If another family member has been diagnosed with GS, this too should be a "red flag "to be tested.

Most people, including some doctors, still equate GS with celiac disease. It is important to understand the difference. About 3 million people in the U.S. have celiac disease but 18-30 million people are estimated to have gluten sensitivity. Celiac disease is a lifelong condition that mandates a strict adherence of a non-gluten diet and should be managed with a knowledgeable physician. GS can produce a low-grade autoimmune reaction and inflammation but doesn't create celiac disease. With GS the body's immune system is stimulated to produce **anti-gliadin antibodies**. Gliadins are prolamin proteins and are a component of wheat gluten. When gluten is allowed into the blood by a loosening of the intestinal lining, the body fights this invader with these anti-gliadin antibodies.

As mentioned in the previous chapter of this book, gluten content in modern wheat is 500 times that found in the wheat cultivated prior to the 1950s and 60's. Why was this type of wheat developed? The simple answers are market demand and world hunger. We think this is a perfect example of the saying "No good deed goes unpunished".

This deed of developing wheat that would address the needs of world hunger merited a Nobel Peace Prize in 1970 to its lead scientist, an American, named Norman Borlaug. His intent was to design a shorter wheat stalk so that the plant would not bend and break as much in the wind and rain. It was modified to become higher-yielding as well. This dwarf wheat, or what we have referred to as modern wheat, is only 2 feet tall. This is much shorter than prior wheat which stood 4 and ½ feet. Dr Borlaug accomplished this feat in only 20 years. There are scientists that say that modern wheat is an example of simple hybridization processes and that plants can naturally modify themselves this way. Our stance is – plants do not evolve naturally into being less than one-half their height and change the amount of gluten in them so drastically in only two decades without aggressive genetic manipulation.

Scientists, even if they are only superficially interested in the subject of agribusiness, know that you cannot take a nutritional staple such as wheat and modify it this drastically without a comprehensive and long-term review of its safety in humans.

Instead, people have been allowed, even encouraged, to eat this new hybridized wheat. Since its inclusion into our diet, a surge in autoimmune disorders and other serious diseases has been noted.

The bio-engineers are hardly done transforming this staple grain. Norman Borlaug wrote in 2000 about how wheat could still be manipulated genetically to produce even higher yield and biotic (e.g. insects) and abiotic (e.g. drought) stress resistance, especially if transgenic wheat was used as parent material. Although, **transgenic** food is not distributed anyplace in the world presently....efforts are being put forth in the world of agribusiness. For example, they would like to **add the genes of cold water fish to wheat so that it could be grown in colder climates. We don't know about you...but fishy wheat hardly sounds appealing and worse, it just sounds wrong.**

3

WHAT IS "LEAKY GUT" SYNDROME?

Dr. Alessio Fasano, head of research at the University of Maryland Celiac Research Center, is credited for discovering the connection between gluten and what is commonly known as "Leaky Gut". In 2000, Dr. Fasano published a paper entitled "**Zonulin** and its Regulation of Intestinal Barrier Function: The Biological Door to Inflammation, Autoimmunity, and Cancer". By writing this paper, Dr. Fasano figuratively blew the "biological doors" off their hinges. He was able to explain how Zonulin, a protein that interacts with the tight junctions between the cells of the intestinal tract wall, could be used as a "biomarker of several pathological conditions, including autoimmune diseases, diseases of the nervous system, and neoplastic conditions." There are multiple mechanisms by which the gut becomes leaky or more permeable and gluten contributes to all of them except physical stress.

The factors that affect the mucosal immune system are:

Dietary Proteins and Peptides

Antibodies

Drugs and Xenobiotics

Physical Stress

Infections

Cytokines

Neurotransmitters

Enzymes

Dr. Fasano discovered that gluten exposure increases the amount of zonulin in the intestinal wall. Zonulin breaks up the **tight junctions (TJ)** between the cells and damages the wall's integrity. This increased permeability is what is referred to as "Leaky Gut".

But that is only the start of the body's troubles. Because of this intestinal barrier dysfunction, all sorts of substances can be allowed to pass through the wall setting off multiple reactions. This partially explains why the symptoms of GS are so varied. Food allergies and intolerance can occur because tiny bits of food, in a form that the body does not recognize, can cross through the intestinal wall. Understand that our food has to be broken down in our digestive system to a point where it can be transferred through our intestinal tract and into our blood to nourish us. When the walls of the intestines become "leaky", food that is not ready to be absorbed into the bloodstream, goes through anyway. The body reacts when it does not recognize a substance. It identifies these unwelcomed invaders as allergens. In other words, we can develop an allergy or intolerance to it.

Ingested proteins, similar to those in our body's composition, are able to pass through a dysfunctional intestinal wall. Our body's immune system identifies these proteins that have passed through the "leaky gut" and can attack them but also can then attack those proteins that are similar in the body's organs and tissues. This is call "**molecular mimicry**". Essentially, the body can start attacking itself which leads to the manifestation of autoimmune disorders.

There is also a defense barrier to keep foreign substances away from our most important organ, the brain. When our immune system has been altered, the blood-brain barrier becomes less viable and neuroautoimmunity may result. This is why any time a patient has GS, a thorough neurological examination of the brain and nervous system should be performed.

Wheat Germ Agglutinin (WGA) lectin has been shown to be able to cross the blood-brain barrier. The conjugated form of WGA enters brain cells by absorptive endocytosis (Pubmed Data: Proc Natl Acad Sci U S A. 1988 Jan; 85(2):632-6, PMID 2448779). Endocytosis is used by all cells in the body to absorb large molecules, such as proteins, by engulfing them. To visualize this more easily, just remember the 1958 sci-fi film, *The Blob.*

Surprisingly, the highest concentrations of WGA lectin are in "whole wheat" bread, including what is considered its healthiest form -sprouted. Sprouting a grain would normally activate food enzymes, increase vitamin content, and neutralize anti-nutrients within the grain. This neutralization does not occur with lectin. Remember from earlier in this book that WGA lectin is part of the wheat plant's defense system against fungi and insects, making it difficult to be broken down. It resists degradation by the same disulfide bonds found in human hair, vulcanized rubber, and feathers. Its use as an insecticide is so desirable, that agribusiness has made WGA-enhanced wheat by way of recombinant DNA technology. So not only was this dwarf, modern wheat designed to have 500 times the amount of gluten, the agricultural scientists decided to magnify the amount of WGA lectin as well.

WGA lectin keeps the plant free of insects but it also may have the potential to produce whole body inflammation in humans.

WGA lectin stimulates the production of pro-inflammatory chemical messengers (cytokines). If you recall, cytokines are one of the factors that produce a hyper-permeable intestinal wall.

It is also believed that WGA lectin is immunotoxic, meaning that it may attach to and activate white blood cells. This can have an adverse effect on the functioning of the immune system leading to an increased incidence or severity of infectious diseases and cancer.

It has already been explained that WGA lectin can pass through into the brain ("the blob" analogy) and what it does to the brain is alarming. We know it may attach to the myelin sheath of nerves and it is also may be capable of inhibiting nerve growth factor (NGF) (PMID: 2720800 Hashimoto S, Hagino A., Dept of Biochemistry, Tohoku Dental University, Japan). Nerve growth factor is critical for the survival and maintenance of sympathetic and sensory neurons. NGF also causes axonal growth and is thought to circulate throughout the body. Our body's homeostasis, our internal equilibrium, can be affected adversely by WGA lectin.

WGA lectin may also be cytotoxic which means it can cause cellular death.

Let's just say….the less WGA we have in our bodies the better……

What else can cause a "Leaky Gut" Syndrome? Actually a number of things, besides gluten and WGA lectin, can disrupt a healthy intestinal lining. Simply aging or intensive exercise can cause the intestines to become hyper-permeable. Stress that affects our psyche can do this as well. Medications that are commonly used can be at fault too. The known medicines, both by prescription and over-the -counter (OTC), are oral antibiotics, anti-acid medications, NSAIDS (Aspirin, Ibuprofen, Naproxen), corticosteroids, and oral contraceptives. Alcohol, caffeine, and lactose (milk sugar) are also at fault. Paprika and cayenne (red) pepper are two widely used spices that can damage the intestinal lining. Sucrose monoester fatty acids are a type of food additive or surfactant that has been shown to significantly affect the intestinal epithelium (PMID: 12673067), The researchers at the Department of Food Science, University of Guelph, Guelph, Ontario, Canada concluded in their results that food additives are responsible for certain allergic types of symptoms and that they can increase the paracellular uptake of food allergens. To round out this list of other factors that contribute to "Leaky Gut" Syndrome, we include gastrointestinal infections from microbes (rotavirus, parasites) and mycotoxins (toxins caused by fungi on dried fruits and stored grain).

We have discussed all the troubles a "Leaky Gut "can cause and how easily the intestinal lining can be compromised. So **here's the good news.** In addition to avoiding gluten products, the intestines can be aided in healing by two things in your spice cabinet. **Black pepper and nutmeg** have been shown to restore Tight Junctions (TJ).

Berberine is another botanical that is thought to "restore barrier function in intestinal disease states." (European Journal of Pharmaceutical Sciences, PMID: 20149867, The Journal of Infectious Diseases, PMID: 21592990). Berberine shows itself to be very versatile in restoring health. It is a nucleic acid-binding isoquinalone alkaloid that has been tested and used successfully in human diabetes mellitus, the cardiovascular system, and displays significant anti-inflammatory activities. Berberine prevents and suppresses pro-inflammatory cytokines. This is the opposite effect of the WGA lectin. The studies showing the positive effects of Berberine are extensive and it appears to be a valuable tool in the treatment of GS.

EPA and gamma linolenic acid (omega 3 fatty acids), **butyrate**, and glutamine have also been shown to heal TJ dysfunctions.

In a recent study, published September 28, 2012 in *Nature*, Chinese and European authors found that patients with Type-2 diabetes have less of the good bacteria that produce **butyrate** in their gut. The scientists also found higher levels of bad bacteria that can cause disease in these individuals.

When intestines have been damaged, the first thing to do is determine which foods need to be eliminated then the intestines need to be "re-sealed" to prevent further damage. Each patient is different with regards to what actions need to be taken for this to take place. Some patients have such a toxic intestinal environment that a special diet needs to be followed before any healing can take place. A knowledgeable doctor in the field of neuro-metabolic or functional medicine should be consulted.

4

IS YOUR HEALTH CONDITION CAUSED BY GLUTEN?

Case Study 1:

A 54 year old female presents with the following symptoms:

Abdominal cramping and bloating

Weight gain

Gastroesophageal Reflux Disease (GERD)

Fatigue

Skin Rash

Chronic neck and midback pain

HISTORY:

Her blood tests for celiac disease are negative. She has been self-treating her heartburn with OTC antacids and has been on thyroid replacement medication for 5 years. Patient reports that she had expected her fatigue to be alleviated by the thyroid medication but has noticed that her loss of stamina persists and is slightly worsening. The patient says she has gained 20 pounds in the past 2 years with no change in her diet or exercise regimen. She states, "If anything, I actually am eating *less* than before but continue to gain weight especially in my mid-section." The skin rash began about 2 years ago and primarily affected her lower limbs. She had sought help from allopathic and holistic physicians to no avail. Corticosteroid cream did help the redness but did not affect the overall "itchiness".

EXAMINATION FINDINGS:

Stool tests were positive for GS. It was explained to the patient that although her stool count for anti-gliadin IgA antibody was 12 units and the normal range is less than 10 units, this did not indicate that she was only slightly sensitive. This test measures the body's reaction to the presence of gliadin in the stool. A number that is above 10 is one of the most reliable indicators for gluten sensitivity. Thyroid tests revealed an elevated anti-TPO antibody indicating Hashimoto's thyroiditis, an autoimmune disease. During the examination, the patient also reported that she experienced chronic neck and upper back pain. A functional chiropractic examination of these areas showed multiple hypomobile cervical and thoracic spinal joints. A thorough neurological evaluation revealed cerebellum dysfunction on the left side evidenced by the presence of dysmetria on the left side during finger to nose testing. Rhomberg sign revealed body sway with imbalance toward the left side.

Treatment:

The patient was placed on a gluten free diet. Two weeks after beginning this diet, the patient reported significant improvement of her abdominal symptoms. She no longer felt the need to lie down after eating. Her stamina had also begun to increase. An OTC antacid, which she had taken daily before going on the GF diet, was used only three times in this two week period. After 4 weeks of care the patient's weight had dropped 12 lbs.

Chiropractic manipulation of the cervical and thoracic spinal joints had alleviated much of her discomfort. Improved mobility within the spinal joints allowed the patient to move her neck more easily and the patient reported sleeping better at night. A physical stressor, such as spinal joint immobility, has an effect on the autonomic nervous system. It has been postulated that manipulation of the spine aids in re-balancing the autonomic nervous system, specifically the sympathetic and parasympathetic subsystems. Patients with over-activity of the sympathetic nervous system may exhibit high blood pressure and excess sweating and inflammation. They exhibit abnormal findings when examining the eyes in addition to other findings. A prolonged physical stressor causes over-activity of the sympathetic nervous system which can lead to disease. Dr. Hans Selye produced a mountain of work on the subject of biological stress and we highly recommend reading his books *The Stress of Life* (1956) and *Stress without Distress* (1974). Another book that deals with the physiology of stress is called *Why Zebras Don't Get Ulcers* by Robert M. Sapolsky. According to the work of Dr Fasano at University of Maryland School of Medicine, physical stressors contribute to the development of "Leaky Gut" Syndrome.

In our opinion, chronic dysfunction of the spinal joints is a type of physical stressor which can contribute to the stress physiology.

Brain-based therapy (BBT) was recommended for this patient. Natural supplements to treat the gut and thyroid were utilized.

The patient reported tolerating the supplements well that had been recommended for her various diagnoses. Her skin rash began to clear after 2 weeks.

The patient described above demonstrated both autoimmune and non-autoimmune diseases.

Case Study #2

A 32-year old male presents with:

Chronic migraines

Constipation

HISTORY:

His migraines are accompanied with vomiting, dizziness, and vertigo. His symptoms began approximately 8 years ago and he has a family history of migraines on his mother's side. These headaches occur 2-3 times per week. He complains of restless sleep and feels that this may be contributing to the frequency of his migraines. He has eliminated known trigger foods such as aged cheeses and red wine from his diet. The patient stated that when he drinks beer, his "chances of having a migraine go way up". He had been prescribed Emitrex but did not like taking it because of the possible side effects of heart attacks and stroke.

EXAMINATION FINDINGS:

Stool tests were positive with a reading of 52 units on the anti-gliadin IgA antibody stool test. He also tested positive for sensitivity to soy. When questioned further about his sleeping, he admitted that his wife complained about his loud snoring and that sometimes she noticed that he seemed to stop breathing. He was referred to a sleep disorder clinic to confirm the diagnosis of Obstructive Sleep Apnea. The clinic conducted a polysomnography study (sleep study) and confirmed the diagnosis. The patient was prescribed a nasal CPAP (Continuous Positive Air Pressure) device. His blood pressure was slightly elevated with a reading of 132/92.

TREATMENT:

The patient was advised to begin a gluten- free diet as well as a soy-free diet. He was educated on the various foods that contain gluten, such as beer. Side Note: There are some commonly available beers that are GF. Anheuser Busch distributes "Red Bridge" GF beer and also provides GF food at Busch Stadium in St. Louis, Missouri.

The patient was placed on supplements that would help intestinal healing with consideration to his constipation. His mild hypertension was monitored. Sleep apnea can elevate the blood pressure of some individuals.

This patient reported that after a few nights of using the CPAP device he felt that he was able to "get into a deep sleep". He experienced one migraine the first week after beginning treatment and two more within the following 3 weeks. He continued to respond well to treatment and his blood pressure readings fell back into the normal range. His constipation has abated. He did notice that if he did consume wheat gluten, he usually would experience a migraine headache within 24 hours.

CASE STUDY #3

A 29 year old woman presents with:

Obesity

Extreme Fatigue

Infertility

HISTORY:

This woman has experienced a gradual increase in weight of 10-12 lbs. per year for the past 3 years. At 5'6" she now weighs 189 lbs. Her previous doctor had refused to test her for GS stating that patients with GS would have intestinal problems. This doctor made a common error in equating GS with celiac disease as discussed previously in this book. Her primary physician had referred her to a rheumatologist after failing to determine a diagnosis for her extreme fatigue. The rheumatologist tested her for lupus and RA but ruled out both diseases. The patient reported that she was unable to perform simple household chores due to her fatigue and usually went straight to bed after work. She could not tolerate Plaquinel (Hydroxychloroquine) that her rheumatologist had prescribed for her diagnosis of "undetermined autoimmune issue". According to the patient, she felt like she had hit a "medical brick wall".

Although she reports an intake of around 1,200 calories per day, she has continued to gain weight. It is often difficult for her to fall asleep at night and awakens frequently after only 4 hours of sleep. Although she and her husband have both been tested for infertility problems, there is no obvious medical reason for their inability to conceive.

EXAMINATION FINDINGS:

A complete blood workup, including tests for thyroid function and cortisol levels, was ordered on this patient as well as a stool test for anti-gliadin antibodies and other food allergens. Physical examination revealed an enlarged thyroid gland.

Thyroid tests showed the presence of anti-thyroglobulin (TG) antibodies and anti-thyroid peroxidase antibodies. A radioactive uptake scan of the thyroid indicated a diagnosis of Hashimoto's thyroiditis.

Cortisol blood levels were found to be slightly elevated. When questioned further about her diet, the patient reported that she would drink coffee and colas throughout the day to combat her fatigue. This habit was strongly discouraged as caffeine can cause an increase in cortisol levels and contribute to her restless sleep pattern and weight gain.

Stool anti-gliadin antibodies (AGA) were elevated at 45 units. The test also showed sensitivity to casein found in cow's milk.

TREATMENT:

The patient was placed on a gluten/dairy – free diet. Supplements, chosen to assist in intestinal, and adrenal healing were recommended. The patient was also advised to discontinue consuming any products with caffeine and soft drinks were eliminated from her diet.

After six months of active treatment, this patient's health had improved significantly. Her weight had dropped to 159 lbs. and she no longer complained of fatigue. She had started working out more vigorously at a local health club. Sleeping through the night was no longer a problem. Cortisol and thyroid antibody levels had returned to normal. Two months after being released from active care the patient phoned the office to tell us the joyful news that she and her husband were expecting their first child the following spring. She was reminded that since GS can run in families, they should have the child tested at 12 months if the baby has any digestive problems or at 18-24 months if there are no symptoms. A breast-fed child should be tested 6 months after being weaned.

CASE STUDY #4

A 6 year old male with Autism Spectrum Disorder (ASD), also referred to as Pervasive Developmental Disorder presents with:

Diarrhea/constipation

Restless sleep habits

HISTORY:

The patient's expressions of ASD were primarily an aversion to making eye contact and repeating words that he hears, a condition termed *echolalia*. He tended to have restless sleeping habits awakening several times each night. His parents reported frequent gastrointestinal problems that alternated between diarrhea and constipation.

EXAMINATION FINDINGS:

NOTE: Although there currently are only limited studies linking ASD with gluten sensitivity, any child who presents with chronic gastrointestinal problems should be considered for GS testing.

Stool tests were performed to determine the presence of gluten and other food allergies. Urine testing for tryptophan was also ordered.

The parents reported that usually one of them would have to stay up with their son until he fell asleep. He had no set bedtime because he would not stay in his bed, preferring to watch television.

The stool tests were positive for both gluten and casein sensitivity. Low levels of tryptophan in the urine were discovered by gas chromatography/mass spectrometry.

TREATMENT:

The patient was placed on a gluten/casein-free diet with supplements to help heal intestinal hyperpermeablity. Tryptophan was also supplemented. The television set was removed from the boy's room. He was allowed to watch the family TV up till 2 hours before "lights out". In the following 2 hours he bathed and both parents took turns reading books to their son.

Initially, little improvement was observed. The parents reaffirmed that they were only giving their son non-gluten and non-casein foods. Only after a thorough investigation into what foods were being consumed, including the brands of foods, was it discovered that one particular soup the child ate almost every other day, did indeed contain gluten. Unknowingly, the parents had allowed the child to eat broccoli cheese soup. Neither broccoli nor cheese contains gluten. However broccoli cheese soup contains *both* gluten and casein. The kitchen habits of the family were also explored in this investigation into why the child was not responding to care. It was discovered that the same toaster was being used to prepare the patient's gluten free bread and regular bread. This is a major source of cross-contamination in the home. After a dedicated toaster was used to prepare only non-gluten bread and the parents made the child's favorite broccoli cheese soup from scratch with gluten free flour and casein-free cheese, their child started to achieve results.

After 6 months of treatment, his gastrointestinal complaints have diminished considerably and his general skin color appears less pale. Although he still has trouble falling asleep, his nighttime awakenings are lessened.

To further boost this autistic patient's immunity, his parents were advised to delete sugar and processed carbohydrates from his diet. Consumption of fresh eggs and high quality meats was encouraged along with probiotics, such as Kefir, and fermented foods.

Given the high correlation of abnormal intestinal permeability in autistic patients (36.7%) and their close family members (21.2%) (Alterations of the intestinal barrier in patients with autism spectrum disorders and in their first-degree relatives PMID: 20683204), it is prudent to have all family members tested. It was found that 2 other family members tested positive for gluten and/or casein sensitivity.

CASE STUDY #5

A 50-year old female presents with a diagnosis of fibromyalgia over the past 10 years. Symptoms include:

Insomnia

Fatigue/malaise

Inability to lose weight

Generalized body aches and pain

Chronic neck and low back pain with chronic stiffness across the upper shoulders

Treatment over the past 10 years has consisted of medications including anti-depressants and Lyrica(pregabalin). A thorough chiropractic and neurological examination with metabolic testing was performed. Functional neurologic testing revealed dysfunction of the right cerebellum. The patient failed several balance tests on the right side. Optokinetic nystagmus testing was decreased to the right side evidenced by diminished pursuit of the eyes to the right and saccade to the left. Saccade refers to the eyes centering back to the left after following an object to the right. The initial pursuit of the object to the right is accomplished by the right parietal lobe of the brain. The right frontal lobe then centers the eyes back to the left after following an object to the right. In this patient her right parietal and frontal lobe activity was diminished. Blood tests revealed anemia, indications of an autoimmune thyroid, and an underactive thyroid. The patient has been on thyroid medication for years with continued symptoms. Further testing revealed gluten sensitivity. It was evident in this case that the patient was having an autoimmune attack on her thyroid gland called Hashimoto's disease. Eating wheat and gluten products will only make Hashimoto's disease worse which was the case with this patient. Treatment was directed at a gluten/wheat free diet, support for the intestinal tract, support for the patient's anemia and brain based therapies to improve the brain dysfunction. Within 12 weeks the patient's symptoms of insomnia, fatigue and malaise were significantly diminished. Her level of chronic neck and low back pain improved. She began losing 3-5 pounds per month.

SYMPTOMS/SYNDROMES THAT MAY BE ASSOCIATED WITH GS

- Abdominal bloating or pain

- Diarrhea

- Constipation

- Flatulence

- Nausea

- Heartburn/GERD

- Fatigue

- Joint pain

- Bone pain

- Mouth ulcers

- Chronic sinusitis

- Autism Spectrum Disorders

- Abnormal menses

- Infertility

- Depression

- Weight gain

- Obesity

- Fibromyalgia

- Headaches, Cluster and Migraine – type

- Chronic Fatigue Syndrome

- Hashimoto's Disease

- Thyroid Disease

- Irritability

- Mood swings

- Body aches

- Gluten Ataxia (loss of coordination)

- Flu-like symptoms

- Numbness

- Peripheral Neuropathy

- Asthma

- Allergies

- Myocardial Infarction (Heart attack)

- Multiple Sclerosis (MS)

- Type 1 Diabetes

- Skin Rash

- "Brain Fog", a cognitive condition

This list, while extensive, is not comprehensive. GS can affect the body by causing wide-spread inflammation as well as allergic and autoimmune reactions. Any organ or tissue can be adversely affected.

If one or more of these symptoms/diseases are relative to you or someone you know, **do not assume that you are gluten sensitive**. See a physician knowledgeable in food sensitivity testing. Not only will this doctor be able to determine the presence of GS, he or she will be able to manage your particular health needs. Every patient's needs are different and thus require an individualized treatment plan.

5

WHICH FOODS ARE GLUTEN-FREE?

Learn to identify food allergies beyond the gluten list that we present in this chapter. Often, a food allergic reaction is subtle rather than a severe life-threatening reaction. Remember that food allergy symptoms can develop in as little as a few minutes to 2 hours after consuming the food.

You can have an allergic reaction the first time you eat a food. It's a good idea to keep a list of foods that aren't tolerated well. How many times have you heard people say "I can't eat that food...every time I do, it feels like my lip becomes numb" or "when I eat Chinese food, it feels like my heart is racing...even when I ask for no MSG (monosodium glutamate)".

Knowledge is power ...knowledge about how your own body reacts to different foods. It isn't feasible for people to be tested for every food, in every combination, with all cross-contamination elements. Look for those subtle and not so subtle hints that your body does not want that particular food.

The mouth is a common area to experience an allergic reaction. It is the just the start of your gastrointestinal system. If a food affects your mouth adversely, then it is logical that it will cause greater problems further along your digestive tract.

The Mayo Clinic lists the most common food allergy symptoms as:

- Tingling or itching in the mouth

- Hives, itching, eczema

- Swelling of the lips, face, tongue and throat, or other parts of the body

- Wheezing, nasal congestion or trouble breathing

- Abdominal pain, diarrhea, nausea or vomiting

- Dizziness, lightheadedness or fainting

Foods that are gluten-free naturally include:

- Meats

- Fish

- Poultry

- Seafood

- Eggs

- Fruits

- Vegetables

- Nuts

- Seeds

- Most dairy products

- Beans

- Olive and fish oils

Foods cannot be breaded or battered-coated unless with gluten-free flour. They cannot be marinated in gluten-containing products like soy sauce unless it too is gluten free.

Grains and starches can also be included in a GF diet. These include:

- Potato

- Wild rice

- Corn

- Buckwheat

- Flax

- Millet

- Rice

- Sorghum (GF beer can be made from this source)

- Quinoa

- Tapioca

- Arrowroot

Gluten free flours can be made from rice, corn, potato and bean. Soy can also be made into flour but we would advise that people make sure, through testing, that they are not sensitive to it.

Some readers may be wondering if oats are among the gluten-free foods. The answers are yes and no. Unless the oat product is labeled "Gluten Free", there is a good chance that the oats have been cross-contaminated with wheat during growing and processing of this grain.

Foods to avoid unless they are labeled "Gluten Free" include:

- Bread and bread rolls

- Pancakes, muffins, biscuits

- Pizza dough

- All bran

- Pretzels

- Gravies

- Cakes

- Pies

- Cookies

- Croutons

- Beer

- Pastas

- Dumplings

- Cereals

- Processed lunch meats

- Rice mixes

- Soups – read labels

- Seasoned potato chips, tortilla chips

- Salad dressings – read labels

- Soy sauce

- Self-basting poultry

- Vegetables in sauce

Foods that can contain "hidden gluten" include:

- Bleu cheese

- Baked beans

- White pepper

- Medications and vitamins using gluten as a binding agent

- Matzo flour/meal

- Malt vinegar

- Some toothpastes

- Hard candy

- Instant coffee

- Licorice

- Curry powder

- Imitation seafood

- Communion wafers (Some churches offer GF versions)

- Some types of chocolate

- Meat and Fish pastes

- Seiten

- Pates

- Some lipsticks

- Brown rice syrup

- Farina

- Chutneys and pickles

- Some sauces

- Not a food, but envelope adhesive makes this list too

Always avoid the following foods:

- Wheat

- Barley (May be eaten if not allergic to this type of gluten)

- Rye (May be eaten if not allergic to this type of gluten)

- Triticale (wheat/rice combination)

- Bulgar

- Durum , often found in pastas

- Graham flour

- Semolina

- Spelt

- Kamut

One last warning...don't eat Play Dough...it has gluten in it......
(But GF versions are sold online) ☺

6

Changing your Gluten Habit / Addiction

Changing the habit of consuming gluten can feel like a monumental shift for some people. This is why we urge households to make this fundamental change together. In the general population, 99% of us who have GS are not aware of it. If another family member has tested positive for GS, there is a greater chance that other members are affected as well.

We have referred to consuming gluten as a habit but there is a fine line between a habit and an addiction. The American Society of Addiction Medicine offers this definition of addiction..." a primary, chronic disease of brain reward, motivation, memory and related circuitry..." They go on to explain "Addiction is characterized by impairment in behavioral control, craving, inability to consistently abstain and diminished relationships."

Anyone wishing to convert to a GF diet must be aware that it may not be an easy transition. What makes "going GF" so difficult is that modern or dwarf wheat has been designed to make it so.

When gluten is digested, it is broken down into peptides. Two of these peptides are called gluten exorphine and giadorphin. With a damaged intestinal wall these two peptides can gain entry to the blood stream and transverse the blood brain barrier. Once this barrier has been breached they can affect the brain by mimicking morphine, an addictive drug. Since gluten can have this effect on the brain, it is considered to be a **neuroactive compound**. These polypeptides have also been called **"gluteomorphins"** referring to gluten and morphine. In essence, modern wheat has been genetically- modified to encourage you to eat more of it. Your habit of consuming breads and pasta is literally "built" into them.

But... habits can be changed.

FIRST STEP

Simply find out if you are gluten sensitive.

Find a doctor who is experienced in functional or metabolic medicine and ask to be tested. Presently, the most accurate way to test for gluten sensitivity is by a stool sample. It can be collected in a specific container in your own home. The stool sample will be tested in a lab for gluten sensitivity but also other common food allergens.

If you suspect that you may be GS, we do not recommend that you go on a GF diet before being tested. Testing will give you a more complete picture if you do suffer from food allergies. For instance, let's say you undertake a GF diet but are also allergic to eggs and soy. You would continue to eat these foods as you are unaware of these allergies. Your chances of seeing any health improvements would be low and you might falsely assume that a GF diet doesn't work for you. Having an objective baseline for your body's allergic reaction will also aid in monitoring intestinal healing.

Having a doctor knowledgeable in this area and who can address each individual's health issues, will increase the prospects of overcoming the debilitating effects of GS.

SECOND STEP

Find out which foods in your house contain gluten.

Go into your kitchen with a red magic marker and place an "X" on all the foods you know contain gluten. Then look at the food labels of the other foods in your refrigerator and cabinets and mark these foods as well.

The Food Allergen Labeling and Consumer Protection Act of 2006 require food labels to clearly identify wheat and other common food allergens in the list of ingredients.

Make a list of all the items you have marked and take it to the grocery or health food store. Replace these items with GF versions. If one store does not have what you need, try another.

Finding GF foods that you enjoy is part of the fun. Some of us prefer pasta made with rice flour and others corn flour and some love flaxseed bread while others prefer breads made with a combination of flours. Brands vary greatly in taste and texture so keep looking to find the brand that you like best…. or you may be inspired to make more food from scratch.

Eating out at restaurants shouldn't be too difficult either. If a restaurant does not have GF meals specified on their menu, ask the waiter if the kitchen can recommend a GF dish. The more times a restaurant have a patron make this request, the more likely they will add GF dishes to their menu. Always ask if the GF food is prepared in dedicated GF utensils to avoid cross-contamination. Meat or egg dishes prepared with no creamy sauces or soy sauce are usually a safe bet as well as vegetables but push the basket of rolls far away. Bread served in restaurants is rarely GF. For dessert, of course you know by now that cake and pie are no-no's, but you can have fruit and most ice creams. Standard ice cream flavors are generally void of gluten but not the "Cookie Dough" flavor. Always look at the ingredients if you are in doubt. According to company data from Blue Bell Creameries, L.P., the stabilizers, emulsifiers, and flavorings in their ice creams are GF too.

THIRD STEP

Breaking the "Gluten Loop"

Gluten, as explained in a previous chapter, can create a physical dependency. Fortunately, this craving can diminish quickly once use is discontinued. Wheat contains a class of addictive substances called opiates so stopping its consumption may be more difficult for some people. This number of predisposed gluten- addicted people, though, is estimated to be relatively small.

By grasping the importance of removing gluten from your diet, you are readying yourself to change your diet and improve your health.

Changing any habit, especially one that has been part of your daily nourishment for most of your life, requires determination. Recognizing the cues - cravings – rewards loop is vital to your success. Finding ways to replace self-destructive foods with healthier alternatives is imperative when one is dealing with GS.

The loop is made up of cues, cravings, and rewards. The cue is you are hungry and it's time to eat, the craving is food, and the reward is your hunger is sated. You only need to change one part of this loop and that is what food is eaten.

Mentally you have to tell yourself that you *are not taking away* foods from your diet...you are *adding* foods.

Let us give an example. Say you like to have pancakes on Saturday morning. This shouldn't pose a problem because GF versions of frozen waffles and pancakes are commonly available in grocery stores. We usually make our own with BisQuick Pancake and Baking Mix. Then again, you may always go out for breakfast so a substitute will most likely have to be chosen. Omelets can easily be made gluten- free, just stay away from the biscuits and toast. Bacon is GF and Jimmy Dean Fully Cooked Sausage Links and Patties are as well. Read the labels of sausage products, though, because some brands do contain gluten. For cereal lovers, the most commonly available is General Mills' Chex Gluten Free line. They come in 6 different flavors including chocolate.

What's for lunch? Turkey and cheese lettuce wraps are great for a simple mid-day meal. Hormel Chili with Beans is GF but *not* the Vegetarian or Turkey varieties. Ordering GF pizza just became easier with Domino's Pizza offering a GF version made with rice flour and starch with potato starch and olive oil. Domino's Pizza does state, however, that it doesn't recommend the crust for those with celiac disease because of the possibility of cross-contamination with gluten.

Dinner is probably the easiest GF meal to prepare. Pastas can be substituted with a GF version. Meat, poultry, and seafood can be prepared without being breaded or battered or you can always use GF flour. Eating out at this time of day is also becoming increasingly easier. Here is a list of restaurant chains that have GF menus or offerings:

Domino's Pizza

Carrabas

Bonefish Grill

Olive Garden

PF Changs

Maggianos

Chances are with more people being tested for GS, the trend for a greater variety of GF foods will continue to rise.

We have discussed the cues (you are hungry or it's time to eat) and the cravings (food). Now let's talk about rewards. The greatest reward will be the restoration of your health and the prevention of more damage to your intestinal wall. Most people find that they are more energetic and less "foggy" when on a GF diet so this is a "reward" in itself. Rewarding yourself with other things besides feeling healthier will complete the loop. Whereas before the "gluten loop" satisfied your hunger or sweet tooth, it caused significant damage to your body. **To ensure that you continue on a GF diet, we suggest that *initially* you reward yourself every day that you are GF.** The rewards can be big or small, you choose. **It is very important to finish the loop with a reward until your GF diet does not take any effort. This is when your brain has re-wired itself with your new habit.**

We would like to review the cues- cravings-rewards loop one more time. You will notice that the only thing that was changed is the craving, which now is a GF food. The reward part is simply amplified to further encourage the brain to remember the new habit.

To encourage your new habit of eating, we recommend that you take the time to develop a menu of what you will eat for a week. This removes some of the effort in sticking with a GF diet. Be sure to add some "treats", such as ice cream or a nice beef steak, during the week especially if you anticipate some hectic times in your schedule. You may want to continue planning your week's diet in advance for several more weeks until choosing GF foods become second-nature.

It also may be helpful for you and others in your household to keep a list of GF foods posted in your kitchen. Be sure to try to keep these items stocked.

Try new GF recipes frequently. We have included several family favorites in this book. Another good source to keep you motivated and to find new recipes and cookbooks is a magazine called Living Without (www.livingwithout.com).

7

GLUTEN – FREE RECIPES & MENUS

We have divided this section into four parts: Breakfast, Lunch, Dinner and Appetizers. At the time of publishing all ingredients were GF but manufacturers sometimes change ingredients without notice. Always check food labels. These recipes have been tested but feel free to improvise. Try to use fresh herbs if possible as they are much more flavorful and healthy for you.

If salt is called for as an ingredient, try using sea salt or coarse kosher salt. Always use freshly ground pepper if possible, remember black pepper is thought to help heal a "leaky gut". Try to avoid aspartame as a sugar substitute.

Be sure to cook all meats thoroughly and avoid cross-contamination with proper kitchen hygiene.

Bon Appétit!

BREAKFAST

Cottage Cheese Pancakes

1 cup   GF Pancake Mix
1/4 cup   Cottage cheese
1 cup   Milk, can also use almond or buttermilk
½ TSP   Vanilla extract (See homemade recipe on page 56)
1-2   Eggs
1/2 TSP   Cinnamon, preferably fresh ground
Butter for greasing pan

Blend all ingredients in a medium bowl.
Ladle ¼ cupfuls onto hot greased skillet or griddle.
Cook until bubbles form then flip.
Continue heating other side until golden brown.
Flip onto warmed platter.
Serve with honey, apple sauce, fresh berries and bananas and/or
Vanilla Sauce (recipe follows)

Makes 8-10 pancakes

SUGGESTION:
Double the recipe and freeze leftover pancakes for an easy GF
breakfast during the workweek.

Pumpkin Pancakes

Substitute 2/3 cup canned Pumpkin for cottage cheese. Add dash of freshly ground nutmeg.
Instead of syrup, try mixing 6 TBS of unsalted, sweet butter with 1-2 TBS of honey.

Vanilla Sauce

2 TBS	Cornstarch
1/3 cup	Sugar – cane, date palm
1/8 TSP	Salt – sea salt or kosher
2 cups	Milk – regular, almond or coconut
2	Eggs, beaten
1 TBS	Butter
2 TSP	Vanilla Extract (recipe for homemade version on Page 56)

Mix cornstarch, salt, and sugar in medium saucepan.
Whisk milk and egg until frothy.
Blend milk mixture into saucepan.
Cook gently over medium heat until mixture comes to a boil, stirring constantly. Do not rush this part. Boil for 1 minute stirring constantly.
Remove from heat and stir in butter and vanilla extract. Serve warm.

Sweet Potato Biscuits

2 cups   Sweet potato mashed, we recommend using canned
1 cup   Sugar (cane, palm, date)
1 cup   GF all-purpose flour
1 cup   Vegetable oil or coconut oil
2 TBS   Baking powder, make sure this is fresh
½ TSP   Ground cinnamon, preferably fresh
¼ TSP   Nutmeg, ground, preferably fresh (helps heal intestinal lining)
Pinch of sea salt or kosher salt

Preheat oven to 375 degrees F.
Lightly grease baking sheets (2) with non-stick cooking spray.
Blend sweet potatoes and oil in large bowl. Add sugar, flour, baking powder, cinnamon, nutmeg, and salt.
Mix well then drop by spoonfuls onto cookie sheets.
Bake 10-12 minutes, checking often until golden brown on bottom.

Makes 16-24 biscuits

Serve with butter, jams/jellies; also great with soups.

Stuffed Apricot French Toast

8 slices	GF bread
2 TSP	GF vanilla extract, divided, see recipe below
1/3 cup	Chopped nuts
8 oz.	Cream cheese, preferably whipped
½ cup	Apricot preserves
3	Eggs
1 cup	Milk, can be regular, coconut or almond
1TSP	Cinnamon
1TBS	Honey (100% organic if possible)
1TBS	Sugar

Pinch of sea salt or kosher salt

In a medium bowl stir together cream cheese, honey, 1 TSP vanilla extract, nuts, and apricot preserves.

In another bowl mix eggs, milk, 1TSP vanilla extract, sugar, salt, and cinnamon.

Divide cream cheese mixture onto 4 slices of bread and top with remaining 4 slices.

Soak both sides of bread in egg mixture then place bread in hot, buttered skillet or griddle and brown on both sides. Repeat.

4 Servings

Serve along with fresh whipped cream (see recipe) and strawberries.

Nutella Stuffed French Toast

Substitute a hazelnut GF spread such as Nutella for the cream cheese mixture.

GF Vanilla Extract

1 liter Rum, Vodka or Bourbon
12 Vanilla beans, split beans lengthwise

Note: All alcohols, if distilled, are GF

Pour off 2 ounces of alcohol from bottle and reserve.
Place beans in the bottle, remember to split the beans first. Place cap back onto bottle and shake. Store in cool, dark place and shake up bottle at least one time per week. After 8 weeks, your vanilla extract is ready.

Fresh Whipped Cream

1 cup   Heavy cream
3 TBS   Powdered sugar

With electric mixer blend cream and sugar together until stiff peaks form. Makes 2 1/3 cups. Refrigerate until served. Well worth the effort!

What is great about making your own whipped cream is that you can customize it. We like to add cinnamon and freshly grated nutmeg in the fall or ground candy cane pieces around the holidays.

Shirred "Cupcake" Eggs

6	Eggs
¼ cup	Milk
3 pats	Butter, unsalted
¼ TSP	Fresh ground pepper
½ cup	Fresh GF bread crumbs
½ TSP	*Salt
¼ tsp	Fresh ground pepper
Muffin Pan	
Cupcake liners	

Preheat oven to 325 degrees F.
Place 6 cupcake liners in muffin pan
Divide bread crumbs into the six cups and press against bottom and sides
Crack one egg into each cup
Add a scant amount of milk onto each egg, not overfilling cup
Add ½ pat of butter onto each egg
Sprinkle pepper and salt on each egg
Bake for 20 minutes or until eggs are set

*There are a variety of salts on the market that can add a distinctive taste to this egg dish. We suggest Oak-Smoked Chardonnay Sea Salt. Sprinkling with fresh tarragon, chopped small, also adds a nice flavor and presentation.

Makes 6 servings

Best Ever Scrambled Eggs

Per Serving:

2	Eggs
¼ cup	Heavy Cream
2 TBS	Butter
¼ cup	Diced Creamy Havarti cheese (optional)

Salt and pepper

Smoothie blender

Whisk eggs and cream with smoothie blender until bubbles appear.
Add eggs to buttered (1TBS) fry pan and cook on low/medium temperature.
Stir often and gently, never "mashing" the egg.
Do not allow eggs to brown
When eggs have set, add 1 TBS butter cut into small pieces
Add Havarti cheese if desired towards end of cooking, allow to melt
Salt and pepper to taste
Serve immediately

Using a smoothie blender aerates the egg producing a lighter, fluffier dish. Adding the butter at the end will help avoid overcooking the eggs.

LUNCH

Cucumber Boats

Per Serving:

1	Whole Cumber peel to create "striped" look
4-6 slices	Turkey, chicken or ham
2 -4 wedges	Garlic &Herb cheese spread
½ cup	Lettuce, chopped
½ cup	Alfalfa sprouts

Condiments

Cut cucumber lengthwise and remove seeds with teaspoon. Stuff scooped areas with alternating pieces of meat and cheese and condiment(s).Top with lettuce and/or sprouts

Either enjoy "open faced" or put one cucumber on the other one to make a "sub".

Substitutions:

Tuna fish salad with olives and green bell pepper

Chicken salad grape halves

Ham and Swiss cheese

CUCUMBER BOATS, continued

Totally veggie – lettuce, tomato, onion, sweet pepper rings, peperoncini, sliced olives

PIZZA

1 ½ cups	GF Pancake and Baking Mix
½ cup	Water
2	Eggs, beaten
1/4TSP	Garlic Powder
¼ TSP	Basil, dried
½ TSP	Oregano, dried
1/3 cup	Olive oil
1 cup	Mozzarella cheese, shredded
¼ cup	Parmesan cheese, grated
¼ cup	Olives- black, green, or both sliced
8 oz.	Pizza sauce
½ cup	Vegetables, sliced (optional)

Pizza Pan or cookie sheet for baking

Preheat oven to 425 degrees F.
Grease cookie sheet or pizza pan
Stir together Mix, garlic powder, basil, and oregano
Add water, oil and eggs. Stir together well
Spread onto pan and bake for 15 minutes
Layer sauce, cheeses, vegetables and olives over crust
Continue baking for 10-15 minutes until cheese melts

4-6 Servings

Lobster Bisque

½ cup	Lobster, cooked and minced
2 cups	Half and Half or milk
1 ¼ cups	Water
3 TBS	GF all purpose flour
2 TBS	Tomato paste
¾ cup	Dry Sherry
1 TBS	Lobster Base

Dash of nutmeg, sour cream or crème fraiche, rosemary sprigs for garnish

Stir all the ingredients except garnishes, into a heavy- duty soup pot over medium heat. Bring to a slow boil while stirring. Simmer for 5 minutes and ladle into bowls. Add a small dab of sour cream or crème fraiche to center of each bowl and dust with freshly grated nutmeg. Add a small sprig of rosemary for an elegant presentation.

Note: The color of the soup will deepen as it cooks. It changes from a bland shade to a rich, almost coppery hue. This dish is best when brought to a boil slowly ...allowing the alcohol in the Sherry to burn off. Some people like a stronger Sherry flavoring but it can overcome this dish's subtle taste. We suggest preparing the dish according to instructions the first time. You can always add more Sherry once it is cooked.

Serve with arugula salad mixed with raspberries, apples, and edible flowers (found at GreenWise Market and other high-end grocers). Dressing is simple: Olive oil and fresh lemon juice

4 Servings

Chunky Chili

3	Garlic cloves, minced
2	Onions, diced
1	Green bell pepper, diced
2 TBS	Vegetable oil
3 TBS	Chili pepper powder (not made from cayenne peppers)
1 TBS	Ground cumin
2 TSP	Ground coriander
1 TSP	Crushed oregano
2 LBS	Ground chuck beef
2 cans	Dark red kidney beans rinsed and drained (15 oz.)
2 cans	Tomatoes, chili-style, diced (14.5 oz.)
1 can	Tomatoes, crushed in puree
2	Limes, cut into wedge

Additions:
Sour cream
Shredded cheese
Green onions, sliced
GF tortilla chips

Heat oil in 5-6 Qt. saucepot then add garlic, onion, bell pepper, and spices. Cook over medium heat for about 8 minutes or until vegetables are tender. Stir frequently.
Add beef breaking it into chunks and continue cooking for 7-8 minutes or until browned.
Add beans and tomatoes.
Heat to boiling over medium-high heat

CHUNKY CHILI, continued

Reduce heat to medium-low and simmer, covered, for 20 minutes. Stir occasionally.
Ladle chili into bowls and squeeze lime wedges over chili. Serve With "Additions" and GF corn muffins (recipe follows).

Makes 12 cups

GF Yellow Corn Muffins

1 cup	Yellow cornmeal
1 cup	Corn flour
¼ cup	Sugar
1 cup	Buttermilk
2	Eggs, beaten
2 TSP	Baking powder
1 TSP	Baking soda
1 TSP	Salt, sea salt or kosher
2 TBS	Shortening, melted
1 can	Green chilies, chopped (7oz) – optional

Preheat oven to 400 degrees F
Grease muffin pan or line with cupcake liners
Sift yellow cornmeal, corn flour, sugar, baking powder, baking soda, and salt together. Stir in beaten eggs, buttermilk, melted shortening, and chilies if desired.
Pour mixture into muffin pan and bake for approximately 25 minutes.

Makes 12 muffin

GF Corn Muffins and Red Tomatoes

Meat-Free & Gluten-Free

1 Recipe   GF Yellow Corn Muffins
4   Large, red tomatoes sliced ¼ in. thick
3   Green onions, sliced

Salt and pepper to taste
Mayonnaise (optional)

Slice muffins in half, place tomato slice on each piece
Top with slices of green onion and mayonnaise (optional)
Sprinkle with salt and pepper

Makes 24 servings

Southwest Jumbo Gumbo

Meat- Free & Gluten- Free

1 jar	Chunky salsa, mild or medium (15.5 oz)
1 can	Black beans, rinsed and drained (15 oz)
1 can	Tomatoes, diced, and in juice undrained (14.5 oz)
2 cups	Water
1 ½ cups	Whole kernel corn, fresh or frozen
½ cup	Rice, long grain white
1 TSP	Oregano
½ TSP	Cumin

Salt and pepper to taste

In a 4 qt. saucepan, add all ingredients, cover and heat to boiling. Reduce heat to simmer for an additional 10-15 minutes or until rice is tender.

Makes 8 cups

Peanut Butter & Banana Sticks

1   Banana, peeled
¼ cup   Peanut butter, crunchy or smooth

Honey for dipping (optional)

Halve banana
Spread with ½ Peanut butter
Dip in honey (optional)

This is a little messy but delicious for a quick, nutritious lunch.

Makes 1 Serving

Cucumber Hearts & Flowers Mini-Sandwiches

1   Seedless cucumber

Wash and cut into ¼ in. slices. The cucumber slices can be cut with small cookie cutters into heart shapes or flower designs or left round. To pack for a "brown bag" lunch, place slices in paper towels then in plastic wrap. Keep cucumber cool. Pack topping separately.

Cucumbers can be used s a base for a number of lunch-time foods. Here are some suggestions:

Tuna salad and alfalfa sprouts
Orange marmalade
Peanut butter and banana with honey
White turkey slices and Muenster cheese
Ham and Swiss cheese
Herbed cheese spread

Serves 1

Tuna on Potato Planks

1 package	Albacore white tuna (6.4oz.)
¼ cup	Mayonnaise
1 stalk	Celery, diced very small
2 large	Baking potatoes, washed and peeled
2 cups	Extra-virgin olive oil

Mix together tuna, mayo, and celery. Refrigerate.
Slice potatoes very thin. Immerse in cold water
Heat oil in large skillet until very hot but not boiling.
Slide half of the potato slices carefully into the skillet.
Cook for about 3 – 4 minutes while gently stirring.
Remove with strainer when golden brown.
Place potato planks on rack and season with salt and pepper.
Repeat with other half of potatoes
When cool, top potato planks with tuna salad.
Serve on platter.

Makes 2 servings

DINNER

Grilled Salmon Burgers with Caper-Dill Sauce

1	Lemon, large
½ cup	Mayonnaise
2 TBS	Capers, drained and coarsely chopped
1 LB	Wild sockeye salmon flakes chopped, or 1 ¼ LB fresh Salmon, skin removed and chopped
4	green onions, finely chopped
¼ cup	Fresh dill loosely packed, chopped
¾ TSP	Salt, sea salt or kosher
½ cup	GF breadcrumbs

Nonstick cooking spray
4 large lettuce leafs

Grate 2 TSP lemon zest then squeeze 2 TBS lemon juice into medium bowl. Add 1 TSP grated peel, mayo, and capers to juice.
In another bowl blend salmon, onion, dill, salt, 1/4 cup GF breadcrumbs and remaining lemon peel.
Shape salmon into four 3 1/2in. round burgers. Press remaining GF breadcrumbs into burgers then lightly spray with nonstick cooking spray.

Place burgers on grill-safe pan on preheated grill. Cook on medium-high heat for 5-8 minutes until lightly browned and internal temperature reaches 145 degrees F.

GRILLED SALMON BURGERS, continued

Serve burgers on top of lettuce with a dollop of Caper-Dill sauce.

Serve with Roasted Beet, Blood Orange & Walnut Salad

Serves 4

Roasted Beet, Blood Orange & Walnut Salad

1 bunch	Beets, trimmed
2	Oranges, blood oranges or navel, remove pith, sliced thinly
½ cup	walnuts, shelled
½ LB	Baby romaine lettuce, or other lettuce mix
½	Red (Bermuda) onion, sliced thinly
2 TBS	Olive oil
2 TBS	Balsamic vinegar or glaze

Place whole beets in microwave safe bowl. Add 1 cup water. Cover with plastic wrap and cook in microwave oven for 6-10 minutes. Let stand 5 minutes. Beets should be tender.
In small skillet, cook walnuts over medium heat 4-5 minutes or until toasted lightly. Stir often. Remove walnuts and chop.
Cut cooked beets into ½ in. cubes
Divide lettuce onto 4 salad plates and top with beets, oranges, onions and walnuts.
Drizzle balsamic vinegar or glaze over plates.

Serves 4

Sunday Shrimp Risotto

8 oz.	Arborio rice, Milanese- style Risotto
2 ½ cup	Water
1 LB	Shrimp, cooked peeled and deveined, wash
2 TBS	Butter, unsalted, divided
1 ½ cup	Peas, frozen
2 TBS	Parmesan cheese, grated

Prepare risotto as directed on package.
When risotto has finished cooking, add shrimp and 1 TBS
butter to pot and cover.
Put peas in a small microwave safe bowl with 1 TBS butter and
cook on high for about 2 minutes.
Add peas and Parmesan cheese to saucepot. Mix well and
serve.

Serves 4

Note: Often, we will make risotto with sodium- reduced
chicken broth replacing most of the water. We also add broth if
the risotto seems too dry.

Beef Stew with Wine
for a larger crowd

5 LBS	Beef, cut into 1 ½ in cubes - don't use stew meat…this dish deserves the best
2 TBS	Butter, unsalted
1 TBS	Salt, sea salt or kosher
½ TSP	Pepper, fresh ground or Montreal Steak
2	Onions, chopped
1 clove	Garlic, minced
3 cups	Red wine, we use an inexpensive Burgundy
1	Bay leaf
¼ cup	Parsley, chopped
1 TSP	Thyme dried, or 1 TSP fresh chopped
3 TBS	GF all –purpose flour
1 can	Tomatoes, diced with liquid
2	Potatoes, peeled and cubed
2 cups	Green beans
3	Carrots, peeled and julienned
1 cup	Garbanzo beans
1 cup	Mushrooms, sliced

Crock Pot

Dry beef cubes thoroughly then sprinkle beef with salt and pepper.
Place in crock pot.
Cook onion and garlic in butter in pan until onion is translucent. Add to Crock Pot.
To Crock Pot add wine, bay leaf, parsley, and thyme.
Cook 3-4 hours on high.

BEEF STEW WITH WINE, continued

Add tomatoes, potatoes, green beans, carrots, garbanzo beans, and mushrooms. Cook for another 3 hours.
When stew is ready, combine GF flour with 1 TBS water to make a smooth paste. Add to hot stew and stir until thickened.

Serve with Creamy Scalloped Potatoes and PERF Salad (recipes follow)

Serves 12

Creamy Scalloped Potatoes

4 cups	Heavy cream
12-14	Large Idaho potatoes, pared and cut into even 1/8 in. slices
3	Garlic cloves,minced

Salt and pepper to taste
Butter for casserole dish

Preheat oven to 375 deg. F
Butter a large, shallow casserole (Use 2 casserole dishes if necessary to accommodate all the potatoes)
This next step should be done in 2 batches.
Using a large saucepan, heat ½ the cream just to the point of boiling over medium high heat. Stir frequently.
Add the sliced potatoes and ½ of minced garlic.
Simmer for 12-15 minutes until potatoes are tender.
Transfer potato mixture to casserole dish
Repeat with second batch adding to casserole dish
Salt and pepper to taste.
Bake for 20 minutes until top is slightly browned.

Serves 12

PERF Salad
(Parmesan, Endive, Radicchio, Fennel)

8-10 oz.	Parmesan cheese, sliced thin (Ask deli to do this if possible)
1 head	Radicchio, cut large pieces
1 head	Endive, cut into large pieces
1 bulb	Fennel (Anise can be used), remove stalk and bottom core, cut into strips
¼ cup	Whole flat-leaf parsley
2 TBS	White balsamic vinegar
1/3 cup	Olive oil
1 TSP	Dijon mustard
1 TSP	Sugar (optional)
Salt and pepper	

Whisk vinegar, oil, mustard and sugar together in small bowl until creamy. Set aside.
Toss salad greens and parsley in bowl with dressing.
Season with salt and pepper
Top with Parmesan slices
Chill and serve

Serves 4

Filet Mignon with Shallot- Red Wine Sauce
for just two

2 TSP	Butter, unsalted
2	Beef tenderloin steaks (*filet mignon*), 1 in. thick, 4 oz each
½ TSP	Salt, sea salt or kosher
¼ TSP	Pepper, fresh ground
1	Shallot, finely chopped
½ cup	Dry, red wine, Pinot Noir recommended
2 TBS	Parsley, chopped
1 cup	Mushrooms, sliced

In a 10 in non-stick skillet, heat 1 TBS butter over medium-high heat until completely melted.

Rinse and thoroughly dry beef. Press salt and pepper into steaks.

Add steaks to pan and cook a total of 10 minutes for medium-rare or until desired doneness. Turning once.

Remove steaks to warm platter.

Add shallots and mushrooms to pan and cook 5 minutes or until shallots start to caramelize. Add wine and heat to boiling. Constantly stir until sauce thickens. Add 1 TBS butter. Stir. Spoon sauce over steaks. Sprinkle fresh parsley over dish.

GF Fettuccine Alfredo

1 LB	GF Fettuccine, we would recommend rice-based pasta
3 cups	Heavy cream
½ cup	Butter, unsalted
½ cup	Peas
1 cup	Parmesan cheese, grated
1/8 TSP	Nutmeg, freshly grated

Salt and Pepper

Cook pasta according to package directions then drain thoroughly.
Heat a large skillet over medium heat then add butter, cream, salt and pepper. Cook till slightly thickened, stirring frequently.
Add peas, cooked pasta, and Parmesan cheese to skillet. Heat until well blended and warmed.
 Place on rimmed platter and sprinkle with nutmeg.

Serves 4-6

Pasta e Fagioli

1 LB	Ground beef, preferably produced with no antibiotics
1	Onion, diced
1	Carrot, julienned
3	Celery stalks, chopped
2 cloves	Garlic, minced
1 can	Tomatoes, diced, preferably with oregano and basil (14.5 oz)
1 can	Red Kidney beans with liquid (15oz.)
1 can	Great Northern beans with liquid (15oz)
1 can	Tomato sauce (15oz.)
1 can	V-8 juice (12 oz.)
1 TBS	White vinegar
1 ½ TSP	Salt
2 TSP	Oregano
1 TSP	Basil
½ TSP	Pepper, freshly ground
½ TSP	Thyme
½ LB	GF pasta, elbow or other smaller type pasta

Brown the ground beef in a large saucepan over medium heat until no longer pink. Drain off most of fat.

Add onion, celery, carrot, and garlic to pan. Sauté for 10 minutes.

Then add remaining ingredients, except the GF pasta. Simmer for 1 hour.

Cook pasta according to package directions. Drain well.

Add pasta to saucepan and simmer for 10 minutes.

PASTA E FAGIOLI, continued

Serve with freshly grated Parmesan, Reggiano Romano, or Asiago cheese.

Instead of salad, serve with a variety of olives, julienned carrots, celery sticks, green onions, peperoncini, and roasted peppers.

Serves 3-4

Crock Pot Beef & Veggie Soup

2-3 cups	Water
2	Onions, chopped
1 LB	Ground beef, browned and drained. NOTE: We always try to use meat that has been humanely raised with a vegetarian diet and no antibiotics or hormones
4 TBS	Beef base
3 stalks	Celery, include the leafy tops
3	Carrots, sliced into small julienned strips
1 can	Diced tomatoes, can be flavored with oregano and basil or plain (15oz.)
½ TSP	Fresh, ground black pepper
1 TBS	Steak sauce, such as A-1
1	Package (16oz) frozen mixed vegetables
½ cup	Butter, unsalted, sweet
½ cup	GF flour

Parmesan grated cheese for sprinkling on at table.

Stir all the ingredients, except the butter and flour, into a crock pot.
Cover and cook for 4-6 hrs on HIGH or 8-12 hours on LOW.
In the last hour of cooking, turn crock pot to HIGH.
Stir together the GF flour and melted butter until well blended.
Add flour mixture to crock pot and stir.
Continue cooking on HIGH until soup has thickened.

CROCK POT BEEF & VEGGIE SOUP, continued

This dish can be made without using any frozen vegetables, of course, just add 2 more cups of whatever vegetables that you like and have on hand...cooked corn, squash, etc. We usually make this dish in the morning when we will be gone all day and using the frozen vegetables helps to save time... but fresh is always better!

We have also prepared this dish without doing the last step of adding the flour mixture. It still tastes great and children love it.

If you want to make it more filling, add ½ cup small GF pasta (We suggest elbow macaroni made with Corn flour). Adjust water amount if needed....or you can add beef broth.

Sprinkle with grated parmesan cheese.

Makes 6 Servings

APPETIZERS

Stuffed Sweet Peppers

1 bag	Mini sweet bell peppers (about 10)
3	Green onions, sliced
3 TSP	Dried cranberries, chopped
1/3 cup	Walnuts, chopped
1 cup	Cheese spread, we recommend garlic and herb

Sauté walnuts at low heat for 5-7 minutes, until they become fragrant. Stir frequently until slightly roasted. Set aside until cooled, and then chop coarsely.
In a small bowl blend, cheese, cranberries, onion, and walnuts.
Cut peppers lengthwise and remove stem and seed.
Fill or pipe each pepper with cheese mixture.
Cover and refrigerate until ready to serve

Makes 20 appetizers

Cocktail Meatballs in Pineapple Sauce

1 can	Pineapple chunks in juice
2/3 cup	Sugar, cane date, palm
½ cup	Rice vinegar
¼ cup	Water
2 TSP	Cornstarch
30	* Fully cooked GF Turkey mini meatballs

In large skillet, stir pineapple with juice, sugar, vinegar, water, and cornstarch until cornstarch is dissolved. Add meatballs and coat with mixture. Cook and cover over medium heat for 12-15 minutes until sauce boils. Can be served in small crock pot to keep warm.

*We recommend Tre Bella Foods GF Turkey Mini Meatballs

Makes 30 meatballs

GF Chicken Nuggets

3/4 cup	GF Pancake and Baking Mix
½ cup	Parmesan cheese, grated
½ TSP	Garlic powder
1 TSP	Parsley, dried
¼ TSP	Pepper, fresh ground
½ TSP	Salt, sea salt or kosher
3 LBS	Chicken, raw strips
3	Eggs, beaten
3 TBS	Butter, unsalted, melted

Dipping Sauce (BBQ, honey mustard)

Preheat oven to 450 degrees.
In paper bowl stir eggs and 2 TBS of water together.
On paper plate blend mix, cheese, garlic, parsley, salt and pepper.
Dip chicken strips in eggs then dredge in flour mixture. Repeat to form a thicker covering on the chicken.
Place chicken strips on cookie sheet. Drizzle butter over top.
Bake for 7 minutes then turn. Bake for an additional 7-8 minutes until chicken has slightly browned.
Serve with your favorite dipping sauce.

Makes 4-5 dinner servings or 12-15 appetizers
Note: Chicken strips can be cut in half when raw to make more appetizer- sized servings

Fruity Brownies to Go

2 Cups of each fruit diced into 1 in. pieces or you can use cookie cutters to make star, flower, etc. shapes out of watermelon and cantaloupe.
-Watermelon
-Cantaloupe
-Strawberries
-Blueberries

1 box GF Brownie Mix prepared as directed, cool then cut into 1 in. squares
Bag of marshmallows
Wooden skewers

Thread alternating fruits with 2-4 marshmallows and 2-3 brownies on each skewer.
Stick skewers into overturned, half watermelon rind that has been trimmed to serve as a stable base. An alternative is to use styrofoam pieces, in a variety of shapes and sizes, that can be decorated for displaying these fruit skewers.

Makes 20+ appetizers

Easy Cheesy Cherry Tomatoes

1 Pint	Cherry tomatoes, large, stems removed
3-4 oz	Cheese, diced into ½ in cubes (try Monterey Jack)

Parsley sprigs for garnish

Place tomatoes stem - side down on cutting board, cut each almost through to bottom into fourths with two cuts.
Place cheese cube into notched area in center of each tomato.
Top with small parsley sprigs.

Makes about 24 appetizers

Shrimp & Bacon Skewers

1 cup	Shrimp, cleaned and cooked
½ clove	Garlic, slice into small strips
½ cup	Chili sauce (We know Frank's Redhot Sweet Chili Sauce is GF)
10 slices	Bacon, uncooked

Small skewers or toothpicks

Mix shrimp and garlic in bowl. Add chili sauce then cover and refrigerate for 3 hours
Cut bacon strips in half. Fry until almost cooked. Remove bacon from pan to cool.
Wrap each shrimp with bacon slice then stick on skewer.
Put skewers on cookie sheet and broil in oven, about 4 inches from heat for 2-3 minutes, turn skewers over after 1 - 2 minutes. Broil until bacon is crispy on both sides.

Makes 18-20 appetizers

Heavenly Deviled Eggs

6	Eggs, 100% organic, large
3-4 oz.	Philadelphia Cream Cheese, softened
¼ cup	Sweet red pepper sauce
2 TBS	Fresh chives, chopped
2 TSP	Dijon mustard
¼ TSP	Salt

Place eggs in a 2 Qt. saucepan with enough water to cover eggs.

Bring to a boil over medium-high heat then immediately remove saucepan from heat. Cover tightly with lid and let stand for 15 minutes.

Drain saucepan and pour cold water on eggs.

Peel eggs under running water.

Slice eggs lengthwise in half. Carefully remove yolks and place in bowl. Stir in cream cheese, sweet pepper sauce, chives, mustard, and salt.

Place egg white halves on serving platter and fill with cream cheese mixture.

Makes 12 appetizers

GF Asian Wings

2 cloves	Garlic, minced
1 TBS	Fresh ginger, peeled and minced
2/3 cup	Green onions, thinly sliced
1/3 cup	Honey
1/4 cup	Hoisin sauce Note: Look for a GF version but be aware that it probably will contain soy
1/4 cup	Soy sauce. Note: Look for a GF version.
2 TBS	Asian sesame oil
3 LBS	Chicken wings

Additions: Celery sticks, carrots, broccoli spears

Place oven rack about 6 inches from broiler
Preheat oven to 425 degrees F
Line broiler pan with foil
In a large bowl stir garlic, ginger, green onions, honey, hoisin sauce, soy sauce, and sesame oil.
Using a sharp knife, separate wings at joint so that you have a "drumstick" and a "thigh". Add wings to sauce. Coat wings well with sauce and let stand for 15 minutes.
Arrange wings on broiler pan and place on already-positioned rack. Bake 25-30 minutes, turning as needed for even browning. Then broil for 5-7 minutes. Watch wings carefully and turn to avoid over browning. Wings are done when glaze thickens and internal temperature reaches 165 degrees F.
Transfer wings to serving plate. Spoon any sauce in pan over wings.

Serve with celery, carrots, and/or broccoli spears.

GF ASIAN WINGS, continued

Serves 6 dinner-size portions or about 18 appetizers.
Have plenty of wet wipes on hand for guests.

Keely's Krabby Kucumbers

6-8 oz.	Crabmeat, fresh or frozen, drained, chop finely
2	Seedless cucumbers, washed and cut into ¼ in slices
½	Kirby cucumber, peel and dice into small pieces
1/3 cup	Mayonnaise
2-3 TBS	Chopped parsley
2 TBS	Chopped chives

Salt and pepper
Parsley sprigs for garnish
Pimentos for garnish

Mix together Kirby cucumber, mayo, parsley and chives in bowl
Add crab to bowl and mix
Season with salt and pepper. Blend well and refrigerate for 1 hour.
Place cucumber slices on serving platter.
Top with refrigerated mixture.
Before serving, garnish with parsley sprigs and chopped pimentos.

Makes about 40 appetizers

Almond Chicken Salad on Cucumber

Nice to serve alongside "Keely's Krabby Kucumbers" for your guests that may not prefer seafood

1 cup	Shredded white chicken breast
¼ cup	Mayonnaise
¼ cup	Sour cream
2 TSP	Tarragon or Rosemary, fresh, chopped
¼ cup	Slivered almonds
¼ cup	Dried cranberries, chopped
2	Seedless cucumbers, washed and cut into ¼ slices

Salt and Pepper

Mix chicken, mayo, sour cream, herbs, cranberries, and almonds in bowl. Season with salt and pepper to taste.
Refrigerate for 1 hour
Arrange cucumber slices on serving platter. Top with chicken salad.

Makes about 40 appetizers

Cucumber slices make a great GF base for a number of appealing appetizers. They also can be used for "Brown bag" lunches in place of bread...just wash and cut into ¼ in. slices,

ALMOND CHICKEN SALAD on CUCUMBER, continued

wrap in paper towels, then in plastic wrap. Keep cool until ready to complete with your favorite topping. See "Lunch" section.

Keegan's Favorite Treat

15-20   Fresh Raspberries
1 small log   Goat cheese

Toothpicks or appetizer spears

Simply stuff each raspberry with a small amount of goat cheese until filled. Pierce each one with a toothpick or spear if serving as an appetizer.

This makes a wonderful treat when packing lunches. Keep cool.

Makes 15- 20 appetizers

Easy Elegant Appetizer

2 heads	Endive, washed
5oz	Herb cheese spread, Note: Perk up store - bought cheese by mixing in some fresh herb like dill
Garnish:	Chopped black olives, alfalfa sprouts

Trim off bottoms of endive heads. Leaves should be about 3 inches long. Make sure leaves are dried.
Place about 1 TSP of cheese spread onto base of each leaf
Place on serving platter
Garnish
Refrigerate until ready to serve

Makes about 20 – 25 appetizers

Smoked Duck Ala Nick Reding

Our good friend and New York Times Best Selling Author has graciously allowed us to include this recipe. We thank him and his family for sharing a truly memorable and entirely delicious hors d'oeuvre. Cheers!

Remove duck breasts, without skin.

Lightly coat each side of breasts with Kosher or other coarse salt.

Let sit for an hour, or until meat is room temperature and salt has begun to work into breasts.

Meantime, soak a handful of hickory chips in beer (GF beer – our insertion).
Smoke duck in an electric smoker at 220 degrees for forty minutes, turning once.

The breasts should be rare to medium rare when they come out of the smoker. Anything beyond medium rare is overcooked! (I do my smoking in batches of 30 breasts, which is as much as my smoker can hold without getting too crowded. Smaller batches will take less time, obviously.)

Let sit for half-an-hour on a cutting board until cooled, slice thin and at an angle. Eat as-is with a heavy red wine, or on crackers (GF- our insertion) spread with raspberry/jalapeno

SMOKED DUCK ALA NICK REDING, continued...

preserves.

Vacuum-sealed, smoked breasts will keep in the freezer for 18 months. Once thawed, smoked breasts can be stored in the fridge for 3 weeks.

8

OUR NEXT BOOK

"BE THE BEST

THE OLYMPIC GLUTEN-FREE DIET"

Preview

In our 30 year plus careers, we have been privileged to work with world-class athletes from a wide range of sports. From football running backs to professional tennis players, we have seen one common link – the most successful players do everything possible to stay healthy.

Nutrition has been a part of athletic training for decades. Only now are we learning that certain foods can adversely affect us physically and mentally. It is not enough to simply consume a well-balanced diet. Foods containing wheat can have detrimental effects on our bodies. Gluten is only one component of modern wheat that can have profound health consequences.

During the 2012 London Olympic Games, several athletes reported that their gluten-free diets helped them to minimize injuries and stay competitive. While some of these athletes suffer with celiac disease and must stay on a gluten-free (GF) diet, others are gluten sensitive (GS) or just feel healthier on a GF diet. They attribute their eating style to giving them that extra edge. These athletes participate in a wide range of sports from pole-vaulting and running to tennis and swimming.

Dana Vollmer, a U.S. Olympic swimmer in the 100-meter butterfly and 200-meter freestyle relay, is a gold medalist in both events and a world record holder. She is the first woman in the 100-meter butterfly to break 56 seconds, clocking in at 55.98 seconds. Her path to Olympic gold was not an easy one. Along the way she had to overcome shoulder, knee and back problems but also a potentially fatal heart condition. On top of these health problems, she would experience stomach aches that would send her to the hospital. The reason for her stomach troubles went undiagnosed and was attributed to stress. Finally, in 2011 she was diagnosed with wheat-gluten and egg sensitivities. Since being on a gluten and egg-free diet, her stomach troubles have subsided. She has said "I feel so much stronger and leaner in the water." according to a *USA Today* article.

Dana Vollmer exemplifies what it take to be an Olympian and successful in life in general. She keeps seeking ways to improve. At the age of twelve, she was the youngest swimmer competing at the 2000 U.S. Olympic trials. Only a few years later, after being diagnosed with Long QT syndrome, she underwent heart surgery to correct the arrhythmia. Still she pressed on. She did not let anything stop her advancement in world class swimming. In 2004, as a 17 year-old, she was part of the team that won Olympic gold in the 800-meter freestyle relay.

During this time she was battling stomach aches that she had experienced since childhood. Only after transitioning to a GF diet did these troubles go away...clearing her way to Olympic gold again in 2012.

Amazingly, all of her physical problems could be at least partially attributed to wheat sensitivity. Modern wheat has components that can disrupt normal intestinal function, produce widespread inflammation causing joint pain, and block essential minerals from being absorbed by the body. Long QT syndrome, the heart condition that affected Dana Vollmer as a child, has been associated with a decreased level of magnesium (Pediatric Cardiology Vol 23, No.1 (2002) Studies of Magnesium in Cong. Long QT Syndrome). Wheat contains two components, phytates and WGA lectins, which can block magnesium and other essential minerals from being absorbed in the body. Although we cannot say that wheat has the potential to cause Long QT syndrome, it is conceivable that it contributes by suppressing mineral absorption.

Olympians require their body to function optimally. They need to absorb all the healthy nutrients they can for their heart, muscles, lungs, and brain. They need to be able to think clearly and not be suppressed by mental or physical stressors. In other words, they have to be the very best at their sport...an Olympian.

In our experience with athletes, having the desire to outperform is the easy part. Many athletes sacrifice normal daily activities for an extra practice session, but few rise to the level of the Olympics. What sets this group apart? The answers will be explored in this book but we will tell you this...**there are Olympic-level athletes**

out there who are having their futures taken away from them by injuries and bodies that could be healthier on a GF diet.

Here's a little background about how we came to be interested in sports and performance. Early on in our careers as chiropractic physicians, we would help a friend who was a trainer at Bollettieri Tennis Academy in Bradenton, Florida. We would evaluate the young athletes and aid with their rehabilitation. Usually, this involved shoulders, ankles, low backs, and elbows/wrists. With the strenuous workout schedules these teens and pre-teens endured, we saw a number of the Academy's students. One of the best players was a 14 year old named Andre Agassi. Believe it or not, he was known on campus for not just his killer serve but for having a great head of hair. Go look at some of his early pictures and you'll see what we mean. One day, after seeing about fifteen strained ankles in a row, Andre walked past us. So we asked the trainer "why don't we ever see that kid?" His answer was "He never gets hurt."

Andre was working just as hard as everyone but everyone else was getting injured. What made that possible? What allowed him to keep working hard and refining his skills while others were sidelined? We can't say what made Andre less susceptible to injury at that time but it is an observation we have seen repeated with other top professional athletes. Any sport's top performers either avoid significant injuries or find ways to heal faster and more completely than their competitors.

One possible causative factor for a predisposition to injury is wheat gluten. Gluten is inflammatory for people sensitive to it. Inflammation has been linked to many chronic disease states and pain syndromes. A gluten-sensitive athlete with repetitive musculoskeletal injuries will not be able to make a complete healing response unless they avoid wheat and "heal and seal" their intestinal tract.

Gluten-sensitive (GS) athletes with chronic inflammation will not see their symptoms subside for any length of time until they clear their diet of inflammation-producing gluten. If the chronic inflammation is not alleviated, they will experience relief from treatment for only brief periods of time. Inflammation from gluten will continue to provoke pain and dysfunction.

World-class athletes put an extraordinary amount of stress on their bodies. They train at their individual sport and cross-train. Each day is structured to mold them into the ideal athlete for their sport. Even their days off are for a purpose. Muscles need time to rest periodically before more strength can be gained.

Having to take time off for an injury is damaging for an athlete in more ways than one. Too many days away from training sets the athlete behind their competitors and their coaches may decide to train others who aren't injured. There isn't any time for sentimentality at this level and the best coaches are always in high demand. Athletes only have so much time to make a name in their sport before those younger and healthier take their place.

Teams will cut players or not re-sign them if an athlete fails to heal quickly after an injury. Years ago, a running back for a professional football team came to us very upset. He had broken his ankle playing and after six weeks of casting was having mobility issues with his foot and ankle. He was afraid that he wouldn't make the team that season...and he was right. We knew that if he couldn't restore the ability to cut sideways across the field, his days with the team were numbered. Fortunately, this story has a happy ending. After only a week of treatment, he made a full recovery and had a successful career. Who knows what would have happened to him if it had taken longer.

Some players aren't so lucky. There's one tennis player that we will always remember. He was only a teenager but he was already experiencing significant low back and hip pain. He loved the game of tennis so much that he would "play through the pain". It was excruciating to see this young man almost in tears following a game, even if it was a game he usually won.

One day, we were observing while Arthur Ashe was evaluating him on the tennis court. This legendary player remarked that our young friend had great potential if only he could move sideways across the court faster. We had talked to his family about how his low back and hip problems would affect his playing ability but they had refused to allow our treatment. They wanted him to only be treated with medication. We hoped, after hearing what Arthur Ashe had said, that his family would reconsider. They didn't, however, and although our friend did rise to being ranked number 12 worldwide, he never became a household name. In our opinion, he was never given the chance to fulfill his potential because his family was not willing to do everything possible to help him become healthier.

We bring up these stories for a reason. Athletes and coaches need to always be searching for ways to advance their abilities, especially when injured or suffering from a health condition. Not every athlete is gluten sensitive but it makes sense to us that *anyone* wishing to be healthier should be tested for GS. It has been estimated and we agree that **99% of those who are GS are unaware of it.**

Each of us has inherent strengths and weaknesses. Olympians simply are stronger both physically and, with equal importance, mentally than the rest of us. This is the reason Olympians have been admired throughout the world since ancient times. We can aspire to be Olympians as children but very few are chosen to actually compete. Still, the goal to be the best is admirable in itself.

As parents, we seek the best life possible for our children. We want them to reach their optimal potential. Whether they have Olympic aspirations or not, we want our children to be smart, athletic, and sociable.

So what's happened?

Our kids are fatter, sicker, and test scores have actually dropped. We all know that childhood obesity has screamed off the charts but it's more than excess weight that is hurting our children – **our kids are really sick!** Parents usually don't have a clue as to what they can do about it. Most of what is written about some childhood diseases, specifically obesity and Type 2 Diabetes, actually blame the parents. We feel this is unfair. We feel....

Parents and their Children deserve a
"Do Over"

The reason we don't blame parents is that almost everyone in the general population, including many doctors, are unaware of the paradigm shift that is occurring in healthcare. Non-celiac wheat sensitivity (NCWS) is, in our opinion, the most under-diagnosed condition affecting the world today. In fact, it was not determined to be a distinct clinical entity until late July 2012. The thought that our food, not to mention a food that is considered to be nutritious, could be harming us is the basis for this paradigm shift. Doctors look at bacteria, viruses, genetics, etc. as being responsible for disease. Now, doctors have to consider genetically-modified food to be a possible source for health conditions, including autoimmune diseases.

Why is wheat suddenly a problem? The wheat we consume today is vastly different from the wheat grown through the 1960's. It has been genetically manipulated to the point that it has been referred to as "Frankenwheat". These changes to the wheat plant are the root of our reasons for writing this book. We will be describing these changes in more detail later but we will tell you this...after reading this book, you will know more about food – triggered disease than the majority of holistic and allopathic doctors practicing today.

What is preventing you from being healthier, slimmer, and stronger? The answer is becoming clearer everyday.

Wheat gluten can:

- Stunt growth

- Cause mid-section fat accumulation and obesity

- Cause intestinal problems

- Provoke allergies

- Cause GERD, heartburn

- Produce depression

- Be suspected of triggering childhood Type 2 Diabetes

- Cause hypotonia (decreased muscle tone)

- Cause vitamin /mineral deficiencies

- Cause inflammation

- Potentially contribute to heart problems

Children with GS, who go on a gluten-free (GF) diet start growing again, lose excessive weight, have fewer intestinal complaints, recover from depression, and generally become more active and mentally happier. This applies to adults as well, with the exception of growing taller.

We have also written a book titled "Wheat Gluten – The Secret to Losing Belly Fat and Restoring Health". It focuses on the elements of wheat that are considered to be responsible for triggering belly fat, a wide range of health issues, and autoimmune disorders. We explain, in easily understood language, what the term "Leaky Gut" actually means as this is an important concept in understanding the widespread damage wheat can cause to the body. It also includes a 3-step plan for transitioning to a GF diet, and over 40 GF recipes.

Wheat gluten sensitivity is poorly understood by most people, including doctors. One of the more common misconceptions is that everyone with GS has intestinal complaints. While bloating and bouts of diarrhea/constipation are common symptoms of GS, many GS-related health conditions are more obscure. For instance, **"brain fog"** is a cognitive condition that causes us to feel tired, have trouble forming our thoughts, be less creative, and generally slower in our thinking. **This condition alone can negatively affect someone athletically, socially, and academically, and in the workplace.**

GS has also been linked to bronchial or lung symptoms, especially asthma. Bronchial asthma can produce:

- Shortness of breath

- Coughing, especially at night or in the morning

- Wheezing

It is very difficult for an athlete to excel in sports, even with medication, if the lungs are suffering from increased secretion of mucous.

The skin can also react to GS. Increased breakouts, eczema, and dermatitis herpetiformis or "gluten rash" have all been connected to GS. "Gluten rash" can occur anywhere on the body, but the most common sites are the elbows, lower back and upper neck, and knees.

"Gluten rash", dermatitis herpetiformis, is one of the itchiest skin rashes known...just think of what gluten can do inside your intestines.

The first thing to do if you suspect gluten sensitivity is affecting you or someone else's health is to be tested. If gluten or other food allergies are detected and have damaged the intestinal lining, it is not enough to simply avoid these foods. The intestines will need to heal and be "re-sealed". A knowledgeable doctor can easily test you for gluten and other food allergies and improve your health naturally with neuro-metabolic medicine.

9

OUR OFFICE IS YOUR GOLDMINE OF INFORMATION

Although our office still makes house calls when necessary, technology has given us the means to combine the personal attention of a house call with the time-saving element of not having to leave your home or office.

Consulting with Dr. Lanzisera can be done in-office or via Skype if traveling is prohibitive and reside in a licensed state.

Our office hosts free seminars on a variety of health issues every month. We discuss diagnosis and natural treatment approaches for a variety of health concerns. A sampling of topics includes:

-Autoimmune conditions, including Hashimoto's thyroiditis

-Weight Loss – A different approach

-Type 2 Diabetes – A growing concern for children and adults

-Fibromyalgia – a chronic condition for many patients

-Migraine Headaches – Solutions to a complex condition

-Chronic spine pain syndromes

-Peripheral neuropathy

Dr. Lanzisera will expand on the complex diagnosis of each condition. He will explain how the body's physiology is interrelated and why dysfunction has occurred. By identifying these dysfunctions, Dr. Lanzisera will explore what natural means can be implemented to help alleviate and improve your condition without the use of drugs and surgery.

Look for the schedule on our web site, WheatGlutenDocs.com, and on our Facebook page or contact the office directly (813) 253-2333. Our toll-free line is 855- DR GLUTEN (374-5883). Reservations are highly recommended.

Periodically, our office will host seminars on Skype. Look for these announcements on our web site and on Facebook or contact our office and we will alert you.

Contact our office to access our new web site with informative videos on a variety of health issues. We are always happy to help you.

813-253-2333

ABOUT THE AUTHORS

Drs. Frank and Lisa Lanzisera are both 1982 graduates of Logan College of Chiropractic. Immediately after graduation they came to Florida to begin their careers. Over the past 30 years, they have treated thousands of patients while staying current with developing technology.

Dr. Lisa Lanzisera has patented an acupressure device designed to help locate acupressure points on the hands and wrists. Her interests are cooking, community involvement, and being a wonky wordsmith.

Dr. Frank Lanzisera received an Associate of Science degree in medical laboratory technology from the State University of New York in 1976. He then graduated with a Bachelor of Science degree from the University of California, Irvine in 1979.

His practice emphasis is a family-oriented chiropractic practice incorporating natural neuro-metabolic medicine for the treatment of acute and chronic health disorders. His interests include sight fishing for giant tarpon with a fly rod.

Professional Papers:

1. Tumefactive Multiple Sclerosis: an Uncommon Diagnostic Challenge. M. Kaeser DC, F. Scali, F. Lanzisera DC, G. Bub DC, DABCN, N. Kettner DC, DACBR. Journal of Chiropractic Medicine, October 8, 2010.

2. Paper presentation on the use of Medx strength testing and rehabilitation of the lumbar spine at the International Conference on Spinal Manipulation in Washington, DC in 1991.

Made in the USA
Charleston, SC
10 November 2014